The Busy Woman's
Guidebook to
Vibrant Vitality

by
Simona Hadjigeorgalis

Acknowledgements

Writing a book, like life in general, takes a tapestry of experiences and people. I'd like to acknowledge and thank the many people that made this book possible.

All of the readers and clients who have taken the journey to Vibrant Vitality have made contributions to my thinking and helped me refine the fuel drop framework to become this Guidebook.

My soul partner and amazing husband Antonios has been instrumental in this project. I'd also like to thank my children, Max and Celia. In addition to the ways they fuel my heart and spirit, they offer continuous motivation for me to prioritize my Vibrant Vitality journey.

I'd like to thank my parents Gail and Larry for all that they've taught me, and for modeling for me what life looks like when we reach for the best parts of ourselves in every aspect of our lives.

Thank you to the people that read early drafts of this book and offered insightful feedback from many perspectives. My parents, my siblings (Scott and Michelle), my life-long best friend Sharon, and my business-accountability partner Arianna.

Thank you to all the people that may not even realize they were offering me cosmic crumbs to follow. Thank you to Mr. V, my daughter's elementary school teacher who asked me to create a fast-and-easy wellness routine for the class; to Matthew H who asked me the powerful question "how can you bottle up what you know so you can have a positive impact on the lives of even more women and girls"; and A.M. from Whole Foods who always offered positive encouragement when I would pick up groceries on my writing breaks.

And finally, if you picked this book up because the cover grabbed your attention, that's thanks to Rupa (also known as libzyyy at 99 Designs). She's a treat to work with.

We all touch each other's live in ways great and small, which is why it's so important that we each let our inner light shine and be seen.

Contents

Preface

Welcome to the Busy Woman's Guidebook to Vibrant Vitality. As you navigate your journey to vibrant vitality, there may be days that you don't have time to read as much as you'd like. That is the sign of your **full life**, and that's **worth celebrating**.

You will benefit from The Guidebook whether you read it for five minutes at a time or if you read a lot all at once. It all counts. Having a full life means that sometimes the only time we have for our own wellness is fitting it in a few minutes at a time in the nooks and crannies of our day. The Guidebook works around your busy schedule and gives you fast-techniques that boost energy in a healthy and body-loving way.

With more energy, there is more time to enjoy your full life rather than be weighed down by it. This is your path to Vibrant Vitality!

Wishes for abundant wellness today and always.

Be Well,
Simona

Chapter One
Navigating Your Guidebook

Imagine having more energy and more time for the things that bring you the most joy and vitality. What would that look and feel like? Would you hop out of bed every morning without an alarm? Who would you be spending your extra time with? Are you up for inviting more **vitality** into your life?

Incorporating the right tiny routines and techniques into your life can make a really big difference in how much energy you have. Unfortunately, the opposite is also true.

When our lives are really busy and we experience modern-stress, if we don't communicate to our bodies that we are safe, then our bodies divert our internal resources as if we were in mortal danger. The way that shows up can be having less energy, less patience, less resourcefulness, and maybe even holding onto a few stubborn and unwanted pound.

The key is knowing which techniques can have the most impact. Let's honor the fact that we are busy, and then focus on how to make the most of whatever moments we do have. It can be challenging to prioritize our wellness when we have so many other things that demand attention. The irony is if we don't prioritize our wellness, we won't have the energy we need to live our busy lives.

Your Guidebook is designed knowing how busy you can get. The information in this book is designed to be bite-sized and designed to work around your schedule.

Why is it just for women?

The Guidebook is an excellent wellness treasure map regardless of age or gender. Yes, there are certainly elements that are universal. However, The Busy Woman's Guidebook to Vibrant Vitality is specifically designed and tailored for women because we have gotten so many messages that tell us it's inevitable that over time our bodies are going to decline and we should just expect that and get used to it.

Well, that's just malarkey!

Yes, our bodies are changing throughout our lifetimes. What worked for us when we were girls will not be the same as what works for us now. That does not mean that we won't be healthy and vibrant. It just means we need a new approach, an approach that fits around our full lives.

In this Guidebook, we will learn how to partner with our amazing human vehicles so we can continue to BE well, LOOK well, and FEEL well throughout our lives.

What can you expect?

Expect to learn how to boost your energy using techniques that were designed knowing how busy you are. Expect tools for healthy and body-loving wellness and vitality. Expect to deepen your connection with your inner wisdom. And expect ongoing Vibrant Vitality.

If you are tired of wondering about the conflicting messages that say eat this not that or workout this way not that way, only later to have the trend change . . . then get psyched. The better we can hear the wisdom of our own bodies, the less we are at the mercy of those external and conflicting messages. You can be vibrant, amazing, and healthy, and look good in those clothes in the back of your closet... without having everything on your plate piling up.

Navigating The Guidebook

Most of the chapters start and end with three fuel drops. The fuel drops represent the key information for fueling yourself for more vitality. Repeating the fuel drops after you've read about them will help you to absorb the information with less effort.

As you navigate your Guidebook, the chapters build upon one another to create a framework that will set you up for continued success long after you've finished reading this book. Your Guidebook also has an appendix. The appendix includes practical tips and applications of the 5 Daily Basics that you'll be learning in Chapter 4.

How many fuel drops do you think you need to embrace to make a difference in your short-term and long-term wellness path? The answer is just one. If you choose to integrate just one fuel drop into your personal operating system you will experience a positive shift in your trajectory towards more vibrant vitality. Effortless wellness and vibrant vitality will become your new wellness set point. Are you up for that?

My own journey to Vibrant Vitality

My own journey to Vibrant Vitality started out of necessity so I could have the energy I needed to juggle (and enjoy!) my hectic life. At 32, I found myself in a position I had never expected to be in. I was getting divorced. Those first few months were challenging to say the least. Besides all that comes along with such a significant life change, I still had my full life to live. I had a demanding job, a wonderful and on-the-move toddler, and I was pregnant.

I needed to stay healthy so I could balance providing for my children and being the nurturing mother they needed and deserved. Through trial and error, I found that abundant energy is fueled by so much more than what we eat. Over the years, I read books, took classes, earned certifications, and attended conferences, about gut health, nutrition, physical fitness, the human mind, philosophy, emotions, Energy Medicine, and healthy energetic boundaries.

As a single working mother, I needed to take what I was learning, and create techniques that worked around my busy schedule. I wanted to be able to fit my wellness around my work and kids (not fit my work and kids around my wellness). When I created methods that worked for me, I'd ask my friends and colleagues to test them too. With practice and experience, I refined my techniques and organized them into this Fuel Drop Framework.

It took me many years to create this methodology, but what it has given me is the gift of enjoying my full life. I went from using sheer will and adrenaline to fuel my busy life, to reaching for my fuel drops and enjoying the journey. Transforming busy into full & vibrant makes a world of difference.

What does my full life look like?

It's still waking up early so I have a head start on the day... but waking up is no longer an alarm set so loud I'll be sure not to sleep through it... NOW on most days I wake up refreshed and ready to hop out of bed and embrace the day.

My days are still full ... but NOW instead of feeling like I am existing on a **giant treadmill of life**, I get to enjoy each phase of my day.

I still occasionally get an intense craving that makes me want to get in my car and drive to the store for a piece of chocolate... but NOW, I usually reach for a fuel drops and when I do, the feeling dissipates and I get to enjoy a healthier relationship with chocolate. *What's your reflexive go to? Sweet, salty, greasy? Something else?*

And it's a good thing I have more time to enjoy my full life, because it's gotten FULLER... the personal p.s. to this story is I am now married to the love of my life. While I am no longer doing this all on my own, I still have a full life and I still reach for my fuel drops.

Exponential Growth

There are a couple of ways you may experience exponential growth. You may hear something that deeply resonates with you. In those moments you'll experience that deep and easy frictionless communication with your inner wisdom. It may feel so easy that you are reluctant to celebrate, but those moments are worth celebrating. I encourage you to be on the lookout for them because when those deep connections lock in, your wellness journey becomes more effortless.

ANOTHER way you might experience exponential growth could be in those friction-filled moments. If you read something that does not resonate with you, especially if it causes friction, we may have uncovered a **wellness blocker**.

When there is noise between your inner wisdom and your conscious thoughts, you don't get to experience all of the energy and vitality that is available to you. Often that noise comes from rules you may have about wellness, or about eating, or about exercise, or about how much time it is "appropriate" to be focused on your own well being. You may not even be fully aware that you have unwritten rules for yourself.

You will learn to identify those rules and notice if they are furthering your wellness journey or inhibiting you from reaching your goals. If you do experience friction, a normal human response will be to want to get out of discomfort. When that happens, there is a possibility that rather than your first reaction being, "Yippee, I just uncovered a wellness blocker", instead you may look externally.

In your very human desire to get out of discomfort, you may get mad at me. That would be a natural initial response. By getting to know me through some of my personal stories, you'll be more likely to notice if that's happening and you'll be able to use that as a reminder to look within for more answers.

Uncovering Wellness Blockers

In those friction-filled moments, consider taking a deep breath and asking yourself what might really be going on. Might there be a wellness rule that you have been carrying around for such a long time that you can now see that the rule no longer makes sense to keep as a rule?

As you bring the discussion into your conscious mind, you can make the choices for yourself that make the most sense for you now. You might choose to tweak or update the rule, or you may choose to keep the rule. Either way, your growth comes when you make clear choices about the rules you keep so they are no longer limiting your ability to hear your body's own inner wisdom. Throughout this Guidebook, you'll learn tips and tools to hear that wisdom even more clearly.

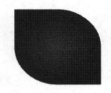

Chapter Two
Your Wellness Destination

This chapter sets the foundation for our wellness journey. The three fuel drops are:

Fuel Drop One: Know Your True North
Fuel Drop Two: Know Why
Fuel Drop Three: Remind Yourself Often

Fuel Drop One: Know Your True North

What is a True North?

True north is a concept that I borrowed from reading a compass. It came from way back in my Peace Corps days in the early 90's before cell phones and GPS systems. The way that I made my way around the mountains to visit the villages where I was working was I had a topographical map and a compass.

Knowing where north was, I could always make my way to where I was going, even if I zigged and zagged along the way. I knew where I was going because I knew the general direction I was walking. That is what our very first fuel drop is all about. It is knowing the general direction where we are going and then honoring ourselves and our **human-ness** to zig and zag in the direction that we want to be going on our wellness journey.

Whether you are going through your Guidebook for the very first time, or you are re-reading it for the 2nd, 3rd, or however many times, it is always important to start with your true north.

Unlike the compass that is somewhat static as north on the compass is an already defined direction... your true north is going to evolve as you do. Our wellness journey shifts and changes as we learn more and as we are in different life stages. Each time you read the Guidebook, start by creating your true north.

In order to find your true north, take a nice deep breath. As you take your deep breath, breathe in through your nose, hold briefly, and then release out through your mouth. Ideally, you'll want to breathe out longer than you breathed in. While you are breathing in, you can think about the nourishing oxygen fueling your cells. Then as you breathe out, release anything that does not serve you as you prepare to do your true north exercise. If you are up for it, go ahead and take that breath now. *Breathe*   Ready to dive into the exercise?

True North Exercise

Preparation

Take a nice cell-nourishing breath. You can do this exercise by thinking to yourself, by speaking to yourself out loud, or by writing your answers... whatever works best for you in this moment.

Exercise Instructions

In this exercise, for maximum benefits, try to suspend your curiosity and answer each question before reading ahead to the next question. If you read ahead, you will still benefit from the exercise, but if you are able to take this one question at a time, you will experience the maximum benefit.

Question 1

Why am I embarking on this wellness journey at this moment in time?

_____

_____

_____

_____

Question 2

Please answer that same question again. "Why am I embarking on this wellness journey at this moment in time?". Before you answer the question again, read your first answer and then ask yourself if that's the complete reason. Ask yourself if there is something more that you want, but you're holding yourself back from saying or even thinking it.

Question 3

Was your answer different between Question 1 and Question 2? Whether is was or whether it wasn't, that's ok. I ask because it is a data point for you. Throughout this book, you are going to be constantly on the look out for data about yourself. Ideally, in the process of learning more about yourself, you'll also learn to see and embrace all the hues of your human-ness and harness the power of that self-awareness. Was your answer different between question 1 and question 2?

Question 4

What are seven things that are going great in your life right now? If you get stuck, start with the basics like access to fresh air and clean drinking water (at least, I hope for you that you have access to fresh air and clean drinking water).

Question 5

List as many things as you can think of to feel grateful for. If you'd like, set a timer and see how many things you can list in two minutes.

What do you feel grateful for?

Question 6

What are you settling for? If you are an optimistic person, that's fantastic, and it most likely serves you really well in most situations. However, there are specific moments in time, like right now, that it makes sense for you to allow yourself to notice what in your life is not how you'd like it to be. What are you settling for? What are you not looking directly at?

Make a list. Dive in. Don't worry, I won't leave you feeling uncomfortable and focused on what you are settling for. But for right now, while you are answering Question 6, really deeply go there. Think about all the places that your life is not exactly as you want it to be, especially in terms of your wellness. If something else comes up for you as you are doing this exercise, allow for those thoughts too.

What are you settling for at this moment?

Question 7

Take a little bit of time to think about each item on the list you just made during Question 6. As you go through each item, ask your inner wisdom if it is something you need to address at this point in time.

If you are writing your answers, circle those you are going to focus on, and draw a simple and clean line through those that you are not going to address at this moment in time. On a clean sheet of paper, write the top one, two, or three things that you really know you are settling for right now and that you know it is time to address.

Question 8

Now that you've noticed you are settling, how are you feeling right now? Are you feeling motivated to do anything differently in your life? What insights have you gleaned so far from doing this exercise?

Question 9

What else might you be able to gain from embarking on this wellness journey at this time? Why is that important to you?

Question 10

In what ways has the "why" that you first wrote down during Question 1 evolved during this exercise (if it has changed)? Did you learn anything from asking yourself the same question more than once?

The Final Step in your True North exercise...

Please take a moment to think back to your lists in Questions 4 and 5 where you focused on what is going well in your life and what you are grateful for. (Or re-read your answer to those questions if you wrote them down.)

Take a moment to really take in your thoughts and joys and let them fuel all the cells in your body. As you are fueling your cells with these nourishing thoughts, consider taking another nice big breath and as you exhale, breathe out anything that is ready to be released as you embark on your journey in the direction of your true north.

Now that you have had the opportunity to really look at your life and why you are here at this moment in time, it's time to think about what your TRUE NORTH STATEMENT is for this wellness journey. Your true north statement begins "I am embarking on this wellness journey at this moment in my life because"...

What's your answer? Why are you embarking on this wellness journey at this moment in your life?

Congratulations on defining your True North! As you continue on your wellness journey, remind yourself regularly of where you are going. And now let's talk about why you are going there.

Fuel Drop Two: Know Your Why

It's very likely that from the true north exercise we just did, you have many thoughts and ideas about why your true north statement is the true north statement that it is. With those thoughts top-of-mind, we are well prepared to dive into fuel drop number two.

There are reasons that this is the moment that you feel motivated and compelled to further your wellness journey. What were those reasons? What ARE those reasons? Know why you are doing this. It is important to know why you are doing this because as you journey through The Guidebook, life will continue to happen. Things will come up.

You are already busy and there are so many other things to pull you away from prioritizing your own wellness. If you are not clear about why you are investing this time in yourself, then those other things will capture your attention until you forget about yourself for a little while.

What I don't want to have happen is you get distracted from remembering this until you find yourself not well. Sometimes, if our body doesn't get our attention when we are well, it will get our attention any way it needs to. It could be having a cold, or worse. So let's focus on being well.

It is not always our fault if we get sick, so please don't add self-blame to your list if you do end up getting sick. However, sometimes getting sick is preventable. So let's focus on our wellness right now and let's remember why we are focusing on our wellness. Why is this a priority for you right now? Why are you going to prioritize your wellness right now? Why are you doing this?

I'd like to encourage you to write out your answer so you can refer back to it. Why are you going to prioritize your wellness right now?

Fuel Drop Three: Remind Yourself Often

Fuel drop number three is to remind yourself often. Right now, while it's fresh in your mind, repeat your true north to yourself and remind yourself why you are pursuing it. What is your true north, and why are you pursuing it?

If you can, remind yourself of that every day, or every week, or every time you brush your teeth. Your true north becomes increasingly more powerful when you repeat it often. For example, you may choose to tie it to brushing your teeth. That choice comes with two benefits. One, it will be easier to remember to do it because you are tying it to an existing habit. And two, you'll probably be in front of a mirror. You can think it to yourself as you look at yourself, or you can say it to yourself as you look at yourself. You can even say it out loud if you want to. Get it into your body so that you know where we are going on this wellness journey and why you are going there.

Fuel Drop Review

Let's take reinforce the three fuel drops from this chapter.

Fuel Drop One: Know Your True North
Fuel Drop Two: Know Why
Three: Remind Yourself Often

Key Take-aways
Your Wellness Destination

As we wrap up Chapter Two: Your Wellness Destination, let's summarize what you just read. Reading the recap of what you just learned, will support your longer-term success in reaching your goals.

Fuel Drop One: Know Your True North
I am embarking on this wellness journey at this moment in my life because...

Fuel Drop Two: Know Why
- Clarity of my motivation will fuel my forward momentum
- Knowing my why will support me on my successful journey

Fuel Drop Three: Remind Yourself Often
- My true north becomes increasingly more powerful when I repeat it often
- I will remind myself of my true north every time I

_____

Chapter Three
The 5 Daily Basics

With our true north fresh in our minds, let's talk about the 5 Daily Basics. We will be diverting from the fuel drop format for just this one chapter. This chapter is more tactical than the rest of The Guide. If you want to streamline your reading, hop forward to *Chapter Four: How We Eat Matters.*

Potent Techniques that Boost Vitality

I've synthesized a few potent routines from this Guide into these 5 Daily Basics. In this chapter, I will introduce you to the 5 Daily Basics. For tips and practical applications of the 5 Daily Basics, check out the Appendix of this book.

The 5 Daily Basics
1. Breath
2. Hydration
3. Harmonizing our energy flow
4. Honoring the digestion zone
5. Rest and repair

How are we going to remember these five things since they are so important? The answer is by chanting them to ourselves. To make it easier to remember, think about this: when you follow these 5 Daily Basics you'll feel awesome...

A-W-E ... double Z, awesome, awesome, awesome are we!

If you are up for it, you may want to chant it. In the audio program, I do an A-W-E-Z-Z cheer. In addition to making the 5 Daily Basics easier for everyone to remember, one of the very fulfilling outcomes of my cheer was getting an email from an audio customer to tell me that her 12-year-old daughter had overheard the cheer and started doing her own version.

What we do for our own wellness matters. It makes a difference in our own lives as well as the people around us.

A: air, or breath, or oxygen

W: water, hydration

E: energy... harmonizing our energy flow

Z: the first Z is for ZONE, that's is honoring the digestion zone

Z: the second Z is for getting enough zzzz's... that's your rest and repair

Let's talk about each of these one at a time starting with A.

A for air, for breath, for oxygen

Taking deep, a cell-nourishing breath is an incredibly powerful tool for your wellness. In addition to being effective, taking a deep breath is a terrific **return on your time investment**.

W for water, for hydration

The W in A-W-E double Z is for water. The second of the 5 Daily Basics is hydration. For optimal wellness, it's important that whatever we are eating, we assimilate or eliminate. Proper hydration aids in both.

E for Energy and harmonizing our energy flow

The E in A-W-E double Z is for ENERGY. As we begin to talk about energy currents in our body, I want you to know that this is not woo-woo mad science.

Studies at credible universities and well-regarded institutes, including Stanford University and the Heart Math Institute are demonstrating that our bodies indeed have energy currents and those currents impact our overall wellness.

One of my go-to techniques for wellness is a 3-minute energy routine, which I've included in the appendix. When we experience modern stress, if we don't communicate to our bodies that we are safe then our bodies will look out for us. One of the ways they look out for us is by diverting resources away from

33

'non-essential' functions. If you had to run from a bear, digestion and metabolism would not be essential. **The 3-minute Routine** is a quick way to communicate to our bodies that what we are experiencing is modern stress, not running-from-a-bear stress.

The first Z is for ZONE. It's about honoring the digestion zone

The digestion zone is the term I coined for that sacred time when our bodies are converting the food we already ate into fuel. Once we eat, our food travels through the digestive tract to be chemically broken down and converted into energy.

What do you think happens when we add more food on top of undigested food? Not a visually appealing thought, but so many of us add more food before we finish digesting what we already ate.

Another way to think about it is this... it's sort of like when you have clothes in the dryer that are almost dry. Makes sense to let them finish drying before you add a heap of wet clothes, don't you think?

The second Z in A-W-E double Z is for ZZZZ's.

Whenever it's possible, get enough of them. Some sources say you can live longer without water than you can without sleep. It is interesting to think about sleep in that category of importance.

Daily Basics Review

Let's go ahead and repeat the 5 Daily Basics one last time to lock them in.

- The A for air reminds us to fuel our bodies with cell-nourishing, stress-busting breaths
- The W for water reminds us to stay hydrated
- The E for energy reminds us to harmonize our energy flow
- The first Z reminds us to honor the digestion zone
- The second Z reminds us to value the restorative gifts of getting enough rest

Chapter Four
How We Eat Matters

Long before we reach our day-to-day choices about what to eat, we've already started a cause in motion.

Fuel Drop One: Our *Meta* Food Choices
Fuel Drop Two: Presentness In Our Meals
Fuel Drop Three: Post-Meal Rituals

Fuel Drop One: Our *Meta* Food Choices

Why a meta perspective? We are going meta so we can gain added perspective about what happens before we reach the moment that we are ready to make decisions about what to eat.

To explore fuel drop one, it may help if you take out your flashlight, your imaginary flashlight that is, because we are going to point a light at some of our automatic decision-making rules about food so we can evaluate and decide what we want those rules to be.

Having rules that run in our unconscious and having the ability to filter is a super useful feature of our minds. If you think about it, it's really quite amazing. If we had to make every single decision consciously with no filters and no rules, we'd never get everything done in our days that we currently get done.

<u>Here's just one example</u>

Take a moment to really think about how many images our eyes take in, and yet, they know what to focus on. Think about that. The challenge is, or perhaps I should say, the cool thing is… we are constantly growing and expanding our perspectives. We know more now than we did when we were kids. Hopefully we even know more now than we did last year at this time. And yet, we all still have some filters, some rules, some automatic decision-making reflexes that we decided upon (or someone taught us) when we younger.

It's helpful to occasionally point a light on those rules and make sure they still apply. What you may find is that there are some rules you love and others that you may want to reconsider. Are you ready to point your flashlight inwards?

Life Safari

We are going to go on a Safari - style adventure. But this one will be one of personal exploration. The direction we'll be aiming for is written in our true north. And the only "danger" we'll be facing will be the danger of not taking the journey at all.

Our younger selves were doing the best they knew how with the information they knew at that time. If we know more now, then we can offer love and appreciation to our younger selves for bringing us to the place that we are now. We can also acknowledge that we have gained some wisdom along the path, which means it's helpful to re-evaluate some of the filters we have for ourselves.

How can we start finding our upstream rules?

Let's start by noticing your recent food choices. As you read through these questions, think about what you have eaten over the last couple of days.

Notice which of these questions seem to apply to you:
1. Were you eating for fuel?
2. As a stress soother? If it was to soothe stress, what triggered the stress?
3. Out of habit?
4. Were you eating for family customs? For example, eating until you need to unbutton your pants on Thanksgiving? Or any number of family traditions around food.
5. For entertainment? To satisfy pleasure? And if you are eating for entertainment or to satisfy pleasure vs. hunger, what is 'enough pleasure' to feel satiated and full?
6. To fill loneliness?
7. To procrastinate?
8. Were you eating to be a good girl and clean your plate? Or, perhaps a good girl and a brave eater who tries new things?
9. To feel connection? Connection with the memory of eating that food at some point in the past? Connection with yourself? Connection with the food on the other end of the fork or spoon?

Answer the questions that resonate with you, and then take it a step further. Ask yourself a follow-up question to your answer … for example, if you answered that you ate to soothe stress, and you say that a work deadline triggered the stress, the next question to ask yourself is 'what would missing a work deadline mean to me'. Ask yourself at least three follow up questions because as you keep asking, you will uncover the deeper cause.

Pay attention to what comes up for you because not looking at those deeper feelings doesn't mean you don't feel them. Your unconscious is feeling them, so you might as well bring them into the light so you can make conscious choices.

Monsters in the Hallway

When I was little, my Dad snored. But I didn't know that. I thought there were monsters and ghosts in the hallways between my room and my parent's room. When I heard the monsterly sounds coming from the hallway, what I'd do is position myself under my blanket in such a way that only my face was showing. For some reason, I thought that if I covered all the rest of my body, including my hair, that the monsters would not see my face even though it was sticking out, which meant I could keep a look out from my made up shield and I would be safe.

Not looking at the deeper feelings is the adult equivalent of hiding from monsters under a blanket. Conversely, when you allow yourself to acknowledge what it actually is that you may not want to be feeling, you might find out, it's not monsters after all. Pointing the flashlight at it may show you what it really is.

It can be scary to look, but what you'll likely find is that you have a better solution by allowing that thought to come into your conscious mind to explore it.

Is there anything standing out for you right now? Have you uncovered any of your unconscious decision making processes? Let's breathe and let those thoughts start to step into the light. As you inhale, breathe in cell-nourishing oxygen. You may also want to picture breathing in light so you can see more clearly. As you exhale, exhale fully. On the exhale, think about releasing any old rules that no longer make sense.

Do you ever fuel your body with non-optimal fuel?

When you fill the tank in your car, do you ever choose sewer water instead of gasoline? Do you ever just keep squeezing the pump after the tank is already full and letting the gas spill down the sides and onto the ground? I am guessing that not only is the answer no, but you may not be able to name a single person that does that to their car.

What about our beautiful and wonderful human vehicles? Ever overfill your body? Ever choose non-optimal fuel? Because you are a human being, I already know your answer.

Fuel drop one helps us do that behavior less of the time. When we look at how we eat from a meta perspective, we get to be more aware of when and why we are doing those behaviors so we can be more conscious about our choices more often. Does that sound reasonable and body-loving to you? If so, you can declare your intentions by reading this out loud:

I choose to be more aware of when and how I am doing the behavior of over-filling my tank AND I choose to be more aware of when and how I am doing the behavior of choosing non-optimal fuel

41

I will pay attention with my conscious mind so that I can see more of my rules so that I can make the choices I WANT to make about fueling my body well

The key to fuel drop one is simply to start noticing. Once we choose to be more aware of when and how we make our food choices, we start to pay attention with our conscious mind more often so we can see more of our rules. When we get curious enough and we choose to point our flashlights inward, we can begin to make the choices we WANT to make about fueling our bodies well.

Fuel Drop Two: Presentness In Our Meals

In the rush of the day, we do not always have time to slow down and be Present as we eat.

Which is more efficient?
- Answer A: multi-tasking ... for example checking email while you eat
- Answer B: sitting with presence and focus on the meal you are eating

Being Efficient

What came to mind when I asked you about being more efficient? Were you thinking about the things that needed to do?

Or were you thinking about the efficiency of your bodily systems that need to convert the food you are eating into fuel to power your brain and your body?

Our bodies put a lot of effort into converting the food we eat into fuel. The digestive process is a mechanical and chemical process that includes our teeth, our saliva, digestive enzymes, and about thirty feet of internal tubing.

By slowing down to be Present as we eat, we are supporting our bodies in the digestive process. Are you willing to prioritize that type of efficiency?

If you think about it, when our bodies are being efficient with digestion, we have the energy we need to do the things we want to do in the post-meal time.

3pm Energy Slump

Do you ever experience the afternoon-crash and feel like you "need" something to perk back up? If so, notice what else is going on. Notice what you ate that day. Notice if you chewed thoroughly. The reason we are noticing is so we can realize that our "efficiency" might actually come from NOT multitasking while we eat.

Sometimes it is not possible to slow down, there is a reason we are busy... we have a lot on our plates. However, there will be moments or meals that you can apply this. And as you do, notice the effect. Notice if you experience an energy-boosting return on your time investment.

Our efficiency and subsequent energy-boost may actually be able to come from carving out some quiet moments to sit, to get present with the food, to notice what we are eating, to honor that we are fueling our bodies, to chew, chew, chew, and to focus some of our attention on the food that is about to nourish us, and on our bodies that are about to assimilate that food into nutrients.

Before we go any farther with this fuel drop, I want you to know that the goal is not perfection. The goal is awareness and conscious decision making. Vibrant Vitality is not about chasing an unreachable "perfectness" in all of our choices. It comes from making body-loving choices more of the time. Does that make sense?

Chewing

Let's talk about chewing a little bit more. Chewing is important because it is the start of the mechanical and the chemical process of digestion. Chewing breaks down your food from the bite you put into your mouth, into the smaller particles that can more easily be digested. If one of the reasons we eat is to fuel ourselves, then it makes sense to give our bodies the best chance at absorbing the fuel.

In addition to starting the mechanical process of breaking down the food, our chewing has a role in the chemical process. As we chew, we are sending signals to the rest of our digestive tract to get prepared for digestion. PLUS, saliva contains digestive enzymes, which means that the longer you chew, the more time the enzymes have to start breaking down the food you are eating. Isn't it cool to notice all the ways our bodies partner with us each and every day. Thank you body!

Another useful chewing tip is to occasionally think about the outcome of your chewing. Remind yourself that you are supporting your body to convert food into fuel. When we step out of our auto-pilot mode and pay attention to details like why we are chewing, it's easier to appreciate (and maybe even enjoy) the process.

Where is your focus at mealtime?

Another way to honor this second fuel drop is to be mentally present at mealtime. One way to do that is to eat at a table. Another possibility is to take a moment to breathe before beginning the meal. The simple act of taking a complete breath may give you the opportunity to 'wake up' from the many thoughts were running through your head and remind your whole self that you are about to sit down and eat.

Gratitude

The third way we can invite Presentness into our meals is with gratitude. There are scholarly articles on the topic of gratitude. There are religious viewpoints on the topic of gratitude. And there are scientific studies on the benefits of gratitude.

If it is comfortable to you, take a moment when you first sit down to eat, and think about what you are grateful for. Those thoughts of gratitude can help transition you from the other parts of your day into the meal and into Presentness with your meal.

Let's take a moment, right now, while we are thinking about gratitude to fill ourselves up so full of gratitude that we are overflowing with it. What thoughts would you need to focus on in order to be over-flowingly full of gratitude? Allow the things that make you feel grateful to enter your mind.

What else fills you up with gratitude?
- What are five small things that fill you up with gratitude?
- What are five big things that fill you up with gratitude?
- What are five totally random and silly things that fill you up with gratitude?

Fuel Drop Three: Post-meal Rituals

Has it ever happened that you finish eating a meal and you are still nibbling? Did it happen after breakfast? After dinner? Every meal? Certain meals? Certain circumstances? When is it easy for the meal to be over when it is over and when is it not so easy?

If your eating does continue post-mealtime, what are you eating (or drinking)? Are you nibbling on a dessert or are you nibbling as you move any leftover food from the pot into the leftover containers?

Do you have any habits such as when you do x you eat y? What's your x? What's your y? Here are a couple of common examples to support you in noticing if you have any automatic rituals: when you watch a show after dinner you eat a pretzel; when you finish the dishes, you drink a glass of wine; after you tuck the kids into bed you eat a cookie.

Do you currently stop eating after mealtime? And if so, is it effortless for you? If it's effortless, Celebrate. You may not realize, but you are in the minority and you may want to tell yourself "I rock". If you don't stop or you do but it's not effortless, that's ok too. You also may want to take a moment to tell yourself you rock. You rock for caring about your wellness enough to read this fuel drop.

Would you be willing to create a new post-meal ritual? One that has you stop eating when the meal is over? One that honors the digestion zone? If that feels too restrictive, would you be willing to create a new post-meal ritual that you implement occasionally?

This third fuel drop is straightforward. Straightforward does not always mean easy. And I recognize that this may take some practice. I also recognize that this suggestion may be bumping up against some of your existing post-meal rituals. Let's just notice that so if any friction comes up either as we are discussing this post-meal ritual or as you go to implement it, we can say -- yeah, an opportunity to see one of my food rules... an opportunity to put on my safari hat and point my flashlight to see what this really means.

Steps for Creating your Post-Meal Ritual

Are you ready to create a conscious post-meal ritual? The first step is to notice when you are finished eating. You can even say it out loud. For example: 'I have finished eating this meal' or 'May everything we just ate become health and harmony within'. How might you want to signal to yourself that the meal is over?

The second step is to consciously enter the digestion zone. The third and final step is to do something to signal to all parts of your mind that the eating time has ended. One possibility is to go brush your teeth.

That's it, three simple steps:
1. Notice
2. Consciously enter the digestion zone
3. Take an action to send yourself a clear signal

Once you have a post-meal ritual, does it mean you have to do it all the time? Like all the fuel drops you are learning here, these are tools in your toolbox and you can use them on your wellness journey as you see fit. As we deepen the connection with our inner wisdom we can look within to know with more clarity what is best.

If you still have some room for being more kind to yourself or more embracing of all your own hues, you are in luck. We'll be doing some exercises in the next chapter to support ourselves on that journey.

Fuel Drop Review

As we wrap up this chapter, let's do what we do, which is to remind ourselves of the three fuel drops.

Fuel Drop One: Our *Meta* Food Choices
Fuel Drop Two: Presentness In Our Meals
Fuel Drop Three: Post-Meal Rituals

Key Take-aways
How We Eat Matters

Fuel Drop One: Our *Meta* Food Choices

- I appreciate my younger self for bringing me to this present moment AND I appreciate the life experience I've had since then that has given me even more wisdom and perspective.
- I evaluate and decide if my food rules are right for me now.
- I make conscious choices to keep, update, or replace the filters and rules I have for myself.

Fuel Drop Two: Presentness In Our Meals

- When I think about being efficient with my mealtime, I'll aim to think about how efficiently my body will be able to convert the food into fuel to power my brain and my body.
- When I practice Being Present with my meals, I am supporting my digestive process.
- Chewing, being present with my thoughts, and gratitude are three ways I can leverage to bring more Presentness to my meals.

Fuel Drop Three: Post-meal Rituals

- I notice when I am finished eating
- I transition from mealtime to post-mealtime using tools including consciously entering the digestion zone and brushing my teeth.

Chapter Five
What Our Minds Are Consuming

The decision about what we are going to put in our mouths is influenced by so many factors. In this chapter, we are going to gain some really powerful tools for noticing when and how we are exposed to messages that influence our decisions about how we fuel our bodies.

The theme for this chapter is What our Minds are Consuming. We'll be looking at how the messages we consume with our minds influence what we eventually choose to consume with our mouths. The three fuel drops are:

Fuel Drop One: External Messages
Fuel Drop Two: Internal Self-Talk
Fuel Drop Three: Our Wellness 5

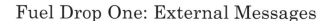

Fuel Drop One: External Messages

Think about what external messages you are exposed to on a regular basis. What messages or triggers are in your current environment? Do you have a bowl of fruit or a pitcher of water sitting in your field of vision? Do you have a bright yellow bag of M&M's sitting in your field of vision?

What's there, subtly or not-so-subtly influencing the ideas that might be popping into your head in the near future seemingly out of nowhere, but actually not truly out of nowhere after all. When you are out and about, do you drive past billboards? Are there brightly colored storefronts inviting you in? Are there fast food signs that set off the quiet hum of their jingle?

In addition to the food messages which you may now be noticing everywhere, what other messages are influencing you? What are the messages you are exposed to in the songs or news or commercials that you listen to? What about when you walk into a store.

Here's another focus I'd like to bring to your conscious attention… what are the images of beauty you are exposed to? Are they real bodies? Are they realistic body shapes? Many times, the images of beauty that we are exposed to are air brushed, altered, literally unattainable because they are not actually real. Think about the non-human proportions of Barbie. Or the non-human eye-shape of the Bratz dolls. What does that do to your self esteem when it is quite literally impossible for you to attain the image of beauty that you are being conditioned to believe?

What about the clothing billboards and magazine ads that we are sometimes exposed to. In addition to being airbrushed, have you ever seen ads with young girls who have not yet fully blossomed into the women they will become? If we dress a girl up like a woman and put her on a billboard or in an ad what is the message about beauty? What do you think happens when you are continually exposed to messages like that? Is it possible that those messages could become noise that blocks your clear and deep connection with your inner wisdom? Who do you think benefits from the conditioned belief tour REAL bodies are not beautiful? That somehow our bodies as they were created are flawed. That our amazing bodies, our beating hearts, our breathing lungs, and our hearing ears are less perfect than an airbrushed and distorted reality.

What would you rather believe about your inner power and beauty? What would you rather believe about your wellness and your inner wisdom? I invite you to sit with that question for a moment and let empowering beliefs about your inner power and beauty flood your mind. Allow yourself to remember how amazing you are. **To remember that you are a beautiful and vibrant being.**

What can we do about all those external messages that are vying for our attention? What if you choose what media you want to consume with the same discernment you choose what food you want to consume? Take note of the messages you are receiving from the radio shows, tv shows, or magazines you currently consume and decide if they are supporting or detracting from your quality of life. Choose consciously. **Awareness is a powerful tool.**

With our eyes wide open to the impact of external messages, let's start noticing the impact of our internal messages as we dive into fuel drop two - internal messages.

Fuel Drop Two: Internal Messages

The good news about fuel drop two is that you are the source, so what that means is that the updates and changes you are choosing to make as a result of reading your Busy Woman's Guidebook to Vibrant Vitality can directly improve the quality of your internal messages.

Since your internal messages are having an upstream impact on the food choices you eventually make, by reading and engaging with your Busy Woman's Guide, you are already on your path towards more effortless wellness. Because our internal messages come in many forms, this fuel drop has three points that we'll be covering. As you read, notice which of the points stirs up the biggest reaction from you. That will help you know which of these points has the most potential to move the needle on your wellness.

When you are observing your reactions, pay attention to the subtle ways your body communicates with you. You may notice a spark of energy OR all of the sudden a feeling of being really tired. You may notice yourself lean in toward your book OR you may notice your mind start to wander. These are all messages. Notice the ways your body language is giving you clues.

Self Talk

Do you ever speak to your body with unkind words? Have you ever gotten angry with your body and called it disgusting?

If you have, I want you to imagine something for a moment. What if you heard someone use that same tone and those same words to talk to their pet or their infant or their elderly neighbor? Can you visualize the words and the tone that you have directed at your body being directed at someone else?

If you had to guess, what type of behavior might you expect to show up in a child that has been told they are disgusting by an influencing figure in their life? If you have ever spoken to yourself with unkind words, what was it about?

One common theme when negative self talk shows up is often around weight loss. As if somehow, if we say enough unkind things to our bodies, those scathing words will scorch off the extra pounds.

When you think about it like that, does the way we speak to ourselves take on a new importance to you? Are you ready to believe that there may be a better approach to communicating with yourself?

If so, get psyched. When we wrap up fuel drop two, we are going to do an exercise to support you in upgrading your self talk. If you already speak to yourself with respect all or most of the time, that's wonderful. The exercise is still for you because it can support you in taking your self-talk to the next level.

Where are your thoughts right now? Whatever you are feeling - it's ok. If you have been unkind or harsh to your body in the past, you can apologize right now and then start being more aware of your self talk. With that awareness, you can make conscious choices to speak to your body with respect. You may even want to start focusing on what is awesome. Hearts that beat every second are awesome. Lungs that breathe whether or not we are paying attention -- awesome. There are so many ways we can celebrate our amazing bodies. It's about what we focus on.

Dancing with our Thoughts and Emotions

Although the Internal Messages fuel drop encourages us be more mindful of how we speak to ourselves, this fuel drop is not about controlling what thoughts pop into our heads. It's about dancing with what comes up. Rather than squashing or controlling or reacting to you thoughts and feelings, try to notice them, try to learn from them. Generally, when we hit a place of discomfort, it's actually a reason to celebrate. It means we may have just uncovered something that could further our wellness.

When you notice thoughts or emotions that make you feel uncomfortable, one thing you may want to consider is taking a nice big breath. Put one hand on your belly and one on your heart and breathe into both hands. Breathe. From that connected place, ask yourself in a non-judging way what the message might be that you are trying to communicate with yourself. Or, ask yourself, what is the rule that you have that makes that thought so unpleasant that you want to control it or squash it.

I am not suggesting that you act on all your thoughts and I am not suggesting that you verbalize all your thoughts. What I AM suggesting is to dance with your thoughts so you see them and learn from them. Leverage them as an opportunity to clear out any noise that gets in the way of your clarity.

When we squash the thoughts we wish we didn't have, we add additional static that interferes with our clarity. We build barriers between our inner wisdom and our conscious decision making. On the flip side, when you acknowledge what you are truly thinking and feeling, you enhance your clarity. It's about getting radically honest with yourself. It's about honoring every hue of your own human-ness. From that place you can more easily and more effortlessly tap into your inner wisdom. How does that sound to you? Are you willing to dance with all of your thoughts? Are you willing to clear out the static that blocks you from tapping into your inner wisdom?

Looking Without

The third and final point we are going to cover in fuel drop two is to notice when you are looking without. Or, to say it another way, notice if you are comparing yourself to another person. How does looking outside ourselves relate to internal talk? It's because when we are looking without, it's not actually a conversation with another person. It's still a conversation with ourselves.

If you find yourself feeling either really good about the way you look or really bad about the way you look based on how another person looks then you know you were just focusing without, and that does not set you up for the highest level of wellness and vitality.

Comparing yourself to others as your measuring stick is a flag for you that you are not focusing within. It is a signal that you have stopped seeking the counsel of your own inner wisdom. The good news is if you notice yourself looking without, you can course correct. When we focus on ourselves and our own choices, we have a greater opportunity to stay in harmony with the wisdom of our bodies.

Have you ever had a commercial jingle stuck in your head? If I say give me a break, what do you think of? A Kit Kat bar? What if I say, I'm a Pepper? What if instead of having someone else's jingle stuck in our heads, we CHOOSE the song in our heads ON PURPOSE? What if the song was full of positive messages? What if the song expanded our wellness and upgraded our self-talk, would you be up for that?

Let's dive into our Fuel Drop Two exercise.

Fuel Drop Two exercise:
Step One: Questions to consider
    1. What are the words you most often repeat to yourself now about your health? Your wellness? Your body shape? Your food choices?
    2. Are they words that most likely expand wellness? If so, what are some additional situations you may be able to sprinkle those word into your regular routine? If not, what are the words or phrases you might want to say more often?

Step Two: Writing your personalized jingle
    1. Think about what messages are important for your wellness path

2. Write them out… free flow with your writing and then you can go back if you want to edit. It does not have to be perfect.
3. Here are a few to get your ideas flowing: I am a beautiful and vibrant being, I value my wellness and vitality, I live a vibrant and well life, I fuel myself on purpose, I treat my human vehicle with love and respect by fueling my body, my brain, and my mind with healthy, vibrant, and energizing fuel.

Step Three: Repetition
1. Repeat your new jingle to yourself often.
2. If you are up for it, record it as a voice memo and replay it to yourself.
3. Any time you notice a commercial jingle "playing" in your head, aim to replace it with YOUR jingle.
4. Any time you notice less-than-positive self-talk, aim to play (or speak, or sing) your jingle to yourself.

Enjoy the experience in the coming days, weeks, and months of what it feels like when the messages you are telling yourself in your own voice are furthering your wellness path!

Fuel Drop Three: Wellness 5

We are strongly influenced by the people we spend the most time with. Fuel drop number three is about noticing our peer group's expectations about wellness and then being conscious about the influencers on our wellness path. Your Wellness 5 are the people that have the biggest influence on your choices about wellness and self-care. Before we dive into our Wellness 5, I want to remind you not to toss out special people in your life, even if you choose not to put them in your Wellness 5. The need for love and connection is part of how we are wired as human beings. There are people in our lives that are rightfully dear to our hearts regardless of their outlook on wellness. Having healthy and nurturing relationships is also important for our wellness.

Laugh, love, and enjoy those special people you have in your life. AND ALSO, at the same time, be conscious of whether or not you want to choose them as your Wellness Influencers. It's about being aware of how our wellness choices are being influenced.

If you realize that there are special people in your life who you are not planning to choose as the members of your Wellness 5 (whether they are family, or close friends, or trusted colleagues, or members of your community) remind yourself what you honor and appreciate about them. It is most likely that you have built your bond on more than wellness philosophy. Accept them for who they are. You can make choices for your own wellness ON PURPOSE, and those choices can be different. Remember, people come in many hues of human-ness. It's not for us to paint someone else's canvas.

That being said, it is for us to paint OUR OWN canvas. When you start to notice, you'll be able to see the many subtle and not-so-subtle ways the people we spend time with can influence us. Be clear who your wellness influencers are and surrounding yourself with positive and wellness-minded messages.

Who are the people that influence your wellness goals right now? Who are the people that you'd like to be influencing your wellness goals? Is there a gap? If so, that's ok. It's just important to notice so you can be aware and so moving forward you can be clear about choosing who your wellness influencers are. I'd like to encourage you to identify five people that you want to consciously choose as your wellness influencers. The first person on your list is likely going to be yourself.

If you don't have four other people in your life right now that fit your idea of who your Wellness 5 needs to be, you are not alone. The good news is you have great instincts. You have already made a choice to spend time reading this Guidebook, which can be a virtual wellness influencer. If you don't have 5 people in your life right now that are a positive influence on your wellness journey, you can create a virtual Wellness 5.

Are you ready to name your Wellness 5? If so, that's great. By declaring your intentions out loud, you are communicating with many different parts of your mind so you can actively move forward with self-harmony and clarity. If you are not ready yet... Yeah, we might have just uncovered a wellness blocker. What might your hesitation mean? Explore it? Notice what comes up. Once you have explored it, even if you don't know who the members of your Wellness 5 are, if you had to name just three people right now knowing you can revise it later, who would those three people be?

Who are your Wellness 5?

1. _____

2. _____

3. _____

4. _____

5. _____

If you don't have four other people in your life right now that fit your idea of who your Wellness 5 needs to be, you are not alone. The good news is you have great instincts. You have already made a choice to spend time reading this Guidebook, which can be a virtual wellness influencer. If you don't have 5 people in your life right now that are a positive influence on your wellness journey, you can create a virtual Wellness 5.

Fuel Drop Review

Let's take a look back on this chapter and a look ahead to what's coming. The theme was What our Minds are Consuming and our three fuel drops were:

Fuel Drop One: External Messages
Fuel Drop Two: Internal Self-Talk Fuel Drop
Three: Our Wellness 5

In the next chapter, we'll be diving into Wellness-Blockers and how to break through them.

Key Take-aways

What Our Minds Are Consuming

In this chapter we gained tools for noticing when and how we are exposed to messages that influence our decisions about how we fuel our bodies. Here are the key take-aways:

Fuel Drop One: External Messages

- I notice what external messages and images I am exposed to
- I aim to choose what media I consume with the same discernment that I use to choose what food I want to consume
- I am grateful for my beating heart, my breathing lungs, and my hearing ears... my REAL body is nature and beauty
- My awareness is a powerful tool

Fuel Drop Two: Internal Messages

- I aim to speak to myself with respect all or most of the time (self-talk)
- I aim to be radically honest with myself
- I aim to honor every hue of my human-ness
- I leverage my thoughts as opportunities to strengthen my connection with my inner wisdom (dancing with my thoughts)
- I focus on my own body and my own choices (looking within)

Fuel Drop Three: Wellness 5

- I consciously choose my Wellness Influencers
- My Wellness 5 includes:

    1. _____
    2. _____
    3. _____
    4. _____
    5. _____

Chapter Six
Wellness Blockers

In this chapter, we'll be talking about Wellness Blockers. By this point, it's likely you have already uncovered a few. It takes practice to remember to link being blocked with celebration, but the more we practice, the easier it becomes. When you hit up against one of your wellness blockers, try to remember to say "Yeah, a wellness blocker".

When we are lucky enough to notice where we are blocked, it's cause for celebration because it means we have the opportunity to break through to the next level of vibrant vitality. The three Wellness Blocker fuel drops are:

Fuel Drop One: Zappers
Fuel Drop Two: The Messages in Cravings
Fuel Drop Three: Mood Altering and Addictive Substances

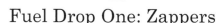

Fuel Drop One: Zappers

There are some common Wellness Blockers and there are also some that are unique to each of us. In this chapter we'll be looking at some of the common Wellness Blockers as well as some fast and effective tools to address them.

How will you recognize your Wellness Blockers?

The clues they offer are different for each of us. For example, if all of the sudden out of the blue you feel like you don't have enough time to finish reading a section you had planned to read, you may have touched upon a blocker. Or you may all of the sudden you find yourself feeling sleepy or resistant. There are many possibilities, so keep paying attention to your body. It will communicate with you when you've hit upon something that may benefit from some inner-exploration.

When you do notice that you've hit up against a Wellness Blocker, if you are up for it, turn your flashlight inward for some inner-exploration. Usually, if you ask yourself enough questions about what it may mean, you'll get to the root cause and have the opportunity to shine a light on the thoughts and rules that are causing friction and possibly creating noise between your inner wisdom and the decisions you make.

Before we dive into our Wellness Blocker fuel drops, I want to remind you that the biggest Wellness Blocker is something we have already talked about. It's when we have become disconnected from our inner wisdom. Stay on the look out for your Wellness Blockers, and when you find them, try to remember to say "Yeah, a Wellness Blocker".

Notice if you experience any of these common zappers, and if so, under what circumstances and how often.
- Negative stress
- Lasting toxic thoughts
- Consistent toxic environment, which can refer to the people you are consistently exposed to or to physical pollutants

- Consistent and debilitating destructive emotions
- Chemicalized foods
- An entirely sedentary lifestyle
- Too much text messaging or too much social media time, and we'll talk about why that's included on this list of zappers

What other zappers come to mind for you right now?

Let's spend some time going deeper with some of these common zappers and then we'll talk about the tools for addressing them. A full life comes with a range of experiences and it is realistic that we will be exposed to some zappers. The key to our abundant wellness is to limit our exposure of those zappers that are within our control to manage; and to use our wellness tools when we confront zappers that are not within our control to manage.

Negative Stress

Let's explore negative stress. Notice I said negative stress. Not all stress is negative. While we are distinguishing between healthy and negative experiences, let's also touch on emotions. All of the emotions can be experienced as healthy or as negative.

Happiness is an emotion that is usually amazingly healthy, but you can be chronically and debilitatingly happy if you force yourself to be happy all the time and don't allow your other emotions to flow naturally and communicate with you. And guilt or anger or envy, which are commonly emotions that we think of as negative, can be healthy if you notice them quickly, seek the messages that your emotions are trying to communicate to you, and take action to restore yourself.

The key is to allow for all of your emotions as they are. To embrace yourself, and all the hues of your human-ness. That does not mean to express or repress every emotion that you experience. It means to notice them and seek the messages.

Stress, for example, is sometimes a word we use when we have other thoughts or feelings attached to a situation. It can be helpful to do some inner-exploration and look for the root cause by asking ourselves questions about what it really means, and being radically honest with ourselves as we answer. Once we see the root cause more clearly, we can aim to solve the way we are experiencing the situation that is causing us stress.

Toxicity

Another common zapper is being consistently exposed to a toxic environment. A toxic environment can refer to the people you are consistently exposed to or to physical pollutants.

If it's coming from the people you are exposed to, it's extra important for you to prioritize your self-care. It may also be helpful to take a deep look at the situation and evaluate what is going on. Is it 100% external, which it very well may be, or do you play any role. If you are contributing, what can you learn from the experience and how can you use those learnings to improve the situation? Also notice if it is a temporary circumstance or if it is something that will likely not change unless you deliberately make a change.

Then decide what you want to do and when you want to do it. It's worth saying that consciously choosing to do nothing is a perfectly reasonable decision sometimes. The key is that it is a decision and not just life happening to you. For all of these zappers, the key is noticing, having a deeply honest conversation with yourself, and then making the decisions that make the most sense for you at this point in time.

Text Messaging

Now let's talk about too much text messaging or too much social media time. Why is too much texting and social media time or even too much unplanned email time a potential zapper? To answer that, let's talk about our brain. The frontal lobe is associated with our creativity, our higher levels of cognition which include problem solving, reasoning, good judgment, and motor function... lots of things we rely on for a Well and Vibrant Life.

When we are checking our phones and social media too often, we are leaving our front brain and operating from our stimulus-response reactions. When we do that on a regular basis, we are essentially training ourselves to spend less time in the front brain.

What can you do? Notice how often you are checking. Notice if you have alerts sounding that communicate to your instinctive response reactions. If you can, turn off some or all of your alerts in the blocks of time your are concentrating. Consider scheduling your social media time, your texting, and emails into specific blocks of time that you designate so you are not reacting.

Counter-Zappers

Counter Zapper One

One really potent Counter Zapper is the 3-minute Routine that I mentioned in the chapter about The 5 Daily Basics. Check out the appendix if you are interested in learning how to do the 3-minute Routine.

Among other benefits, the 3-minute Routine is a tool for working in harmony with your body's inner wisdom. Our bodies' are really wise and there was a time in our human history that our negative stress and other zappers were a signal that we were in mortal danger.

The 3-minute Routine helps us to communicate to our bodies that what we are experiencing is modern stress.

Counter Zapper Two

Another tool that you've already learned is the **A** in A-W-E-Z-Z. Taking a deep, cell-nourishing breath is a fast way to counter a zapper. When we are experiencing zappers, we sometimes unconsciously begin to take shallow breaths. Investing twenty seconds to take a deep breath can have a noticeably positive impact on our physiology, our mental and emotional clarity, and our mood. Breathe.

Counter Zapper Three

I'd like to teach you one more really great tool. It's a foot massage. Be prepared for this one. Although many find it to be an effective counter-zapper, it's not one of those relaxing types of massages.

Use your thumbs to rub the top of your feet in those soft channels between the bones of your toes. It might hurt the first time you try it so as with everything in this Guide, listen to your inner wisdom to determine what's right for you.

What you'll likely notice is that if you do this massage for yourself, you'll feel a sense of decreased tension in your entire body. You may even be able to notice the feeling of toxic energy leaving your body. Sometimes when we have experienced a toxic emotion or have been consistently exposed to a toxic environment, some of the emotions or feelings, or what I am referring to here as toxic energy, gets trapped in our bodies. This top-of-foot massage is a great tool for setting it free.

We just talked about some of the common wellness zappers and three really effective tools for supporting your wellness when you experience zappers.

Those tools are:
1. The 3-minute Routine
2. A for Air, for deep cell-nourishing breaths
3. The top-of-foot massage

Fuel Drop One Exercise

Having a full life means you are going to experience some zappers, so let's do an exercise to prepare you to manage those zappers in a way that best supports your Vibrant Vitality.

First... make a general list of wellness zappers. If you are writing your list, it will be help to fold your piece of paper vertically. Use the left-hand column to list as many Zappers as you can think of.

_____ _____
_____ _____
_____ _____
_____ _____

Next, use the right-hand column to answer the following questions:

- Which of those Zappers do you currently experience either right now, or on a regular basis
- Is the Zapper within your control to manage
- If so, what can you do to manage it? When are you going to do that?
- And/ or if not, what tools are you going to use to support your wellness in these situations... when are you going to use them?

Fuel Drop Two:
The Messages In Our Cravings

The way we communicate with our cravings can either be a path towards even greater wellness or it can become a Wellness Blocker. To make our discussion on cravings bite-sized and designed for optimal absorption, I've chunked this fuel drop into two sections: lifestyle-related and nutrient-related cravings. Cravings come in more than the two categories we'll be talking about here. What I'd like to encourage you to do as you read through these two categories is to notice what you can learn and apply to cravings in general.

Lifestyle-related cravings

A great place to start this discussion is with the palindrome desserts and stressed. Desserts is stressed spelled backwards, which I hope you find to be a memorable way to remember fuel drop two which is the messages in our cravings.

We'll be talking about mood altering substances in fuel drop three, but let's just briefly touch on that topic right now in the context of cravings. Try to notice when you are being drawn to desserts with a goal of altering your mood out of discomfort (for example eating as a very temporary band aid when you are feeling stress).

If you are not a dessert craver, that doesn't mean to tune out. We started with desserts because of the memorable palindrome, but we could substitute the word desserts with treats of any kind (salty, greasy, and more). So even if it's not desserts you turn to in stress, if you turn to food when you experiencing negative stress, then you may have a lifestyle related craving.

Stress and Cravings

If you do find yourself in a situation that you are craving treats, try to notice, then ask yourself questions. I am not suggesting that enjoying a treat is a sign of stress. And I am not suggesting that every time you want a treat it means you are having a food craving. I am also not suggesting you restrict yourself from eating treats. What I AM suggesting is that you notice when you are craving foods and you pay attention to what else is going on. Aim to notice if the message in your cravings is really a communication from your wise and loving body asking you to take care of yourself.

What can we do to combat stress-related cravings? The 5 Daily Basics is a great tool for lessening the grip that stress-related cravings can sometimes have. If doing some but not all of the 5 Daily Basics is what works best for you, do it without guilt and without 'shoulding' all over yourself. These are tools to support you, they are not meant to restrict you or add undue pressure.

Another tip for combating a stress-related cravings is sauerkraut. A bowl of sauerkraut can sometimes instantly nip a craving, so if you like sauerkraut, it's worth a try.

Sleep and Cravings

Another common culprit of lifestyle related cravings is lack of sleep. It's common because so many of us have a lot on our plates. Often times, as we try different options for finding the right balance for ourselves, one of the aspects of our lives we typically experiment with is our sleep since it accounts for so many hours of each day.

On the one hand, that's great to experiment and see what the ideal amount of sleep is for your body. But chances are if you are getting less sleep it's not for an experiment, it's more likely because of things that you are juggling right now in your fully engaged life.

Often times when we cut back on sleep we'll notice cravings the next day. Or if it's chronic lack of sleep, we may notice that it impacts our food choices in general. If lack-of-sleep is the root cause of a craving, getting in more sleep (or a 20-minute power nap) can help. It's not always easy to juggle everything so finding the time to get in a full night's sleep can sometimes be challenging, but it's really worth considering. One tip for clearing up time so you have the hours available to get enough sleep is to make quality decisions about where to say no.

Cravings and the Food-Memory Connection

Let's talk about happy memories associated with food. Taste is a powerful sense. What happens for some of us, some of the time is that we are having an amazing time and while we are having that amazing time, we happen to eat something specific... and boom, we may have just linked the smell and taste of that food to the memory of all the positive feelings we are having in that moment.

You can't taste being on the receiving end of a twinkling smile. You can't taste feeling the warmth of the sunshine on a beautiful day. You can't taste so many of the amazing experiences life offers us. Which means, if we happen to be eating something while we are in a heightened state of enjoyment... guess what.... sometimes we mistakenly link up that food with all the other positive feelings we were experiencing in that moment.

Can you think of anything you crave somewhat regularly even in times when you are well rested and not in negative stress? Once you have that food item in your mind, notice... is there a memory associated with it? Was there a time or multiple times that you were eating that food and experiencing something non-food related with your other senses?

If you do find you have linked up a happy memory with food, take a moment to think about all of the joy in that memory. Enjoy the whole scene. What was going on? What are some of the details that are standing out for you? What else? Isn't it cool the way that memory can bring back so much happiness just by thinking about it consciously and focusing on it. Now, while we are remembering that time, let's really notice... was that food we linked up the true cause of the happy feelings we were having and are having now as we remember that time? Or was it all the other things going on as we were eating the food? List the other things now.

Noticing the way that food item was linked to a wonderful memory may help loosen the craving. You don't need to eat the food you were eating that day to feel the joy you were feeling during that experience.

Nutrient-related cravings
Sometimes our cravings are our wise and loving bodies letting us know we need a nutrient. Our environment is changing over time. The foods we do and do not have access have changed over time. For example, we can now leverage transportation to enjoy fresh produce all year round, even those of us that live in places that get cold and snowy in winter.

Unfortunately, not all the changes are for the better. One example of that is that some of the soil our food is grown is less full of nutrients than it once was, which means some of the produce we are eating has had less of an opportunity to absorb soil nutrients. The reason that may be causing some of your nutrient-related food cravings is because we used to be able to get more of our trace minerals from a bigger variety of the foods we ate.

What can we do? You are actually already doing the biggest thing you can do. You are deepening your connection with your inner wisdom and you are clearing out the static and noise that can block your ability to fully tap into that inner wisdom. By strengthening your ability to hear and correctly interpret what your body is asking for, you are already far along your path.

What's the message?

Paying attention to the messages in our cravings can help us hear what our bodies are trying to communicate to us. For example, a common cause of chocolate cravings is your body asking for magnesium. If you find yourself craving chocolate, you may find it worth it to experiment with eating some magnesium-rich foods like spinach or cashews.

Cravings Log

A great tool you can use to further your internal communication is start a cravings log. If you do experience cravings, try to notice them. And then try to investigate them. You can ask yourself questions and get curious. If it helps you remember to do it, picture going on another Safari - style adventure and this time, rather than pointing our flashlights towards finding our hidden wellness rules, we can point the flashlight towards understanding the messages in our cravings.

Questions to consider when a craving arises:
- What else is going on for me right now - internally or externally
- Do I have any memories associated with eating this particular food I am craving
- Have I craved this before, and if so how often do I crave it and when do I crave it
- Am I getting enough sleep
- Am I hydrated
- What time of year is it
- What time of day did I have the craving
- Where am I in my menstrual cycle
- What did I eat today and when
- What did I eat yesterday
- Have I been moving my body regularly
- What other questions might you want to ask yourself?

Cravings quick-check

As we wrap up fuel drop two, let's review some of the questions we can ask ourselves when we encounter cravings.

1. What else is going on for me right now?
2. Do I have any strong memories associated with eating this?
3. Could this be a message from my body letting me know I need something else in my diet?

Try to keep an eye out for the messages in your cravings. Whether you start to keep a log of when and what you are craving, or you simply notice and ask yourself questions. Remembering that the craving can be a message for you to interpret may change the power that craving holds over you.

Fuel Drop Three: Mood Altering and Addictive Substances

We know that drugs and alcohol are mood altering substances and we make choices to use or not use those substances armed with that awareness. However, we don't always remember that food is a mood altering substance.

One of the most important messages I'd like to convey with fuel drop three is to raise your awareness and encourage you to notice when and if you are reaching to food to change your mood. If you do find yourself in that situation, consider evaluating what you want to do and make a conscious decision to use or not use food in that way.

How do you know when you are reaching to food to alter your mood? Ask yourself questions. Notice what else is going on for you. Ask yourself questions such as 'what does this mean for me'. Dig deeper with your answers by asking follow up questions such as 'what else might this mean'. As you keep staying curious and you keep staying radically honest with yourself, you generally find the answer that gives you more clarity.

It sounds straight forward, but you and I both know that it's not when it comes to food. Do your best to ask yourself questions that inform the choices you make about what, why, and when you eat. Be kind and loving to yourself. Allow yourself the room to stumble as you are figuring this out. The good news is that the more you deepen your connection with your inner wisdom, the more intuitive these choices become.

Big Food

Do you know the food industry spends a mind boggling amount of money on research to determine what will get your attention, what will entice you to take that first bite, and what will keep you coming back for more.

If you think about it from a macro perspective for a moment, so much of our food supply is managed with the objective of giving you a product that you will buy, that will last a long time so it can make it to your pantry without spoiling, and that will make a profit. It's gotten to the very upsetting point that some foods are being designed to be enjoyable but not satiating so you eat more of their product. Even when they are not purposefully designed to circumvent your body's innate wisdom, when we are eating nutrient-poor foods, we can be eating plenty and still legitimately hungry because we are not being nourished.

What can you do?

You can read the labels on the food you are buying and making informed choices. Even if you are buying your food from a more nutrition-conscious food market, it's still helpful to read the labels.

The bummer of it is, it costs more to eat real food than the chemicalized food-like substances we are being offered everywhere we turn. Fortunately, as we start fueling our bodies with more nutrient-dense foods, what we may find is that we don't need to eat the large portion sizes that our culture has been training us is normal. As we decrease our portions back to normal sizes, even if it's only for some of our meals, that helps with our food budgets.

What do you think? Are you willing to read your food labels so you can make informed and conscious choices about how you are fueling your body? If so, when are you going to start? Are you going to start with the food that is currently in your pantry? Are you going to start with everything you buy moving forward? Visualize when and what you are planning to do.

If not, that's completely ok. It's your choice to make for yourself. If you have decided that now is not the right time to start reading labels, it may be helpful for your to do a little inner-exploration to make sure you are making your decision with clarity. Consciously choosing to do nothing is a perfectly reasonable decision sometimes. The key is making that decision from a place of clarity.

Before we wrap up fuel drop three, let's talk about soda, and particularly diet soda, because even though it isn't food, soda does impact the way we eat and can be quite disruptive to our wellness.

If soda is currently part of your daily routine, you may want to consider experimenting with how you'd feel if you spent three days without it. What would you drink? Could you substitute it with water? Or maybe you'd prefer the water if you jazzed it up with an ice cube and a slice of lime? Might you be willing to give it a try? Whatever you decide, decide what is right for you at this point and then visualize what you are going to do and when you are going to do it.

As we wrap up fuel drop three, let's do a quick review:

We talked about raising our awareness about when we are using food as a mood altering substance and noticing the circumstances so we can learn and make conscious choices moving forward.

When we do notice ourselves engaged in the behavior of turning to food as a mood altering substance, we have an exercise for asking ourselves questions so we can further deepen our connection with our inner wisdom.

We talked about reading the labels on everything we eat or drink

Fuel Drop Review

In this chapter we talked about Wellness Blockers and our three fuel drops were:

Fuel Drop One: Zappers
Fuel Drop Two: The Messages in Cravings
Fuel Drop Three: Mood Altering and Addictive Substances

Enjoy the process of uncovering your Wellness Blockers. When you do find a blocker, try to remember to say 'Yeah, a Wellness Blocker'. That can signal to your mind that it's something that can benefit from self-reflection.

Key Take-aways
Wellness Blockers

When we notice our wellness blockers we get the opportunity to address them. If you find yourself hitting up a against a blocker, try to remember to celebrate… "Yeah, a wellness blocker".

Fuel Drop One: Zappers
- I aim to notice when I am experiencing a zapper
- I aim to limit my exposure to zappers that are within my control to manage
- I use the counter-zappers when I am faced with a zapper that is not within my control to manage

Fuel Drop Two: The Messages in Cravings
- I aim to notice if the messages in my craving are actually a form of communication from my wise and loving body
- If I am experiencing cravings, I aim to remember that I have body-loving tools available to me such as the 5 Daily Basics
- I ask myself questions, such as:
  - What else is going on for me right now
  - Do I have any strong memories associated with eating this

o Could this be a message from my body
letting me know I need something else in my
diet?'

Fuel Drop Three: Mood Altering and Addictive Substances

- I aim to notice if I am reaching for food to change my mood
- If I do reach for food to change my mood, I evaluate what I want to do and make a conscious decision to use or not use food in that way
- I aim to be kind and loving to myself
- I am understanding of myself when I zig and zag

The Power of Repetition

Before we continue forward in the direction of your true north, let's briefly notice where we just came from. Taking one step at a time in the direction of our dreams can take us further along on our journey than we may realize. Occasionally, it's worth it to pause and celebrate how far we've come!

This repetition is another one of those tools that sets us up for success. The most potent tools can take less time than we think, and they have a really big return on the time invested. Are you up for reinforcing what you've already learned and setting yourself up for your next level of vibrant vitality?

As we look back on the first chapters, enjoy the experience. If there is anything you didn't try, or any exercises you haven't yet done... try not to put undue pressure on yourself. You can choose to go back or you can keep pressing ahead and trust that the information you are taking in is supporting you in deepening your connection to your inner wisdom.

Do your best, and that will always be enough. And remember, guilt and negative stress do not support your highest wellness. My suggestion is you read this recap to deepen what you have learned, not to evaluate if you have done enough. Let's start with a wonderful cell-nourishing breath. Ready? Let's do that now.... inhale and then fully exhale. Breathe.

Now that your cells are fed, take a moment and think about the first three things that come to mind about the material you've already read. No pressure on yourself, whatever answer you come up with is what you need to know at this moment in time. Ready? Let's do that now, what are the first three things that come to mind?

Wasn't that interesting? Sometimes the three points that pop into our heads are the obvious ones and sometimes what pops up is a little surprising. But it's always a useful exercise! The next question I have for you is: What is your true north? With your true north fresh in your mind, let's review all of the fuel drops you've already learned.

Your Wellness Destination
    Know your True North
    Know Why
    Remind Yourself Often

The 5 Daily Basics
A - W - E - Z – Z
    Air (breath, oxygen)
    Water (hydration)
    Energy (harmonizing our energy flow)
    Zone (honoring the digestion zone)
    ZZZ's (rest and rejuvenation)

How We Eat Matters
    Our *Meta* Food Choices
    Presentness in Our Meals
    Post-meal rituals

What Our Minds Are Consuming
    External messages
    Internal self talk
    Our Wellness 5

Wellness Blockers
    Zappers
    The Messages in Cravings
    Mood altering and addictive substances

Isn't it cool to realize how much you have already learned? Are you noticing shifts and new tiny habits that are pointing you in the direction of your true north? What choices have these fuel drops inspired for you so far?

_____

_____

_____

Would you be willing to choose one thing from what you've learned so far and commit to doing it today? If so, what one thing did you choose? _____

Chapter Seven
Human Vehicle Basics

Our bodies are fueled on much more than just the food we eat. In this chapter, we'll focus on the foundational fuel for our human vehicles as we continue to build a sturdy and lasting wellness foundation.

Fuel Drop One: Nourishing our Cells
Fuel Drop Two: Nourishing our Hearts
Fuel Drop Three: Rest and Rejuvenation

Before we dive into fuel drop one, let's talk about eating and movement for just a moment. I want to mention them because, they are important, and we will be talking about those topics later in this Guidebook.

We receive so many messages that tell us if we want to be healthy and vibrant we have to eat certain foods or move a certain way. Yes, those things are important; but to create lasting change, it's important to build on a sturdy foundation. That's why we are layering our fuel drops and creating a framework that sets us up for long-term success.

Human Vehicle Basics

Think back to a time when you were a little kid and you were playing in the moment with all of your heart. Notice what it felt like. Or think back to a time that you were in new love and your belly was full of excitement and love.

Chances are, the focus was on feeling totally alive and present, and chances are, even though food wasn't the top priority at the moment, you were probably not hungry because you were fueled with foundational fuel.

With that in mind...

Fuel Drop One: Nourishing Our Cells

In fuel drop one, we are going to talk about three ways we can nourish our cells with breath, hydration, and energy hygiene. If additional ways of nourishing your cells feel important to you, that's great! Our goal with fuel drop one is to point our focus at nourishing our cells, so if you want to take another path to reach that outcome go with it.

Nourishing our Cells with Breath

Take a normal breath right now as you are reading. Notice, are you exhaling for at least as long as you are inhaling? Are you shallow breathing or taking deep breaths?

Place one hand on your chest and one hand on your upper stomach (above your belly button and below the ribs) right now. Notice what part of your body is rising when you breathe normally. Are both hands rising? One or the other? What else do you notice?

If taking cell-nourishing breaths is already easy and instinctive for you, celebrate. You are among a minority of modern-day adult human beings, and surely your body appreciates all those gorgeous daily breaths.

If it's tough for you, you are not alone. It just means we have some work to do. And when I say you are not alone, know I am talking from personal experience, and I can tell you **it does get easier**.

I can still remember this mini-story I am about to tell you vividly. Even though it's a tiny story, almost so tiny it seems unimportant, and even though it was years ago, it made a lasting impression on me so I'll share it with you.

I was sitting in my car after work, still in the parking garage. I was about to put the keys in the ignition, and then I stopped and thought to myself, I don't remember the last time I took a breath.

I had a quick conversation in my head about the urgency of time and the need to get to childcare before pick up time. I knew logically it would only take 20-seconds, but I really felt like choosing to take that one breath could make me late. It was challenging to trust my logic, but I decided to invest 20-seconds in myself and take a deep breath.

As I consciously breathed in, I could not get the breath to go down further than my chest. I had been stressed all day gunning for a deadline and running from meeting to meeting, and somewhere along the way, I must have started

95

shallow breathing. As I sat there, I started to wonder when I had last taken a full breath.

I don't know if it had been hours or days or longer. What I do know is it took quite a bit of intention to make the choice to prioritize that one breath.

When I finally treated myself to the breath, I could feel the stress from the day start to leave my face and my body and I literally felt the spaces in my body open up to allow for wellness to flow more freely.

When I think back on that moment, I still feel like my entire body appreciates that I chose to take that breath that day.

One of the beautiful things about our bodies is they take care of us as best they can, even when we are not taking care of ourselves. So let's take a moment to acknowledge that and thank our bodies. Thank you body!

I can tell you a few things from that experience:
- It's worth it to keep on practicing. One minute of conscious breathing is an amazing thing you can do for your overall wellness (or even one single conscious breath if that's all you can prioritize at the moment)
- The more often you remember to practice taking deep, cell-nourishing breaths, the more likely you'll be to take full breaths even in the moments you are not paying attention

- It WILL get easier over time. We were born knowing how to breathe fully. Just watch a baby breathing and you'll see the amazing and natural way they use their diaphragms. We can get back there.

More likely than not, it will not be as easy as you'd expect it to be the first few times, keep on keeping on. It will be worth it. If you find yourself feeling like you don't have time for wellness, remember that the simple act of breathing consciously can really make a difference in how much energy you have.

Breathing Techniques

Let's talk about a few breathing techniques. Try them out and see which you like best. Or, if you already have a breathing technique you enjoy, go with that. The important thing is to fuel your cells with oxygen.

For all the techniques we are talking about here, the inhale is through the nose. To remember that, think about your anatomy, our noses have filters inside them. Isn't it cool to remember that those nose hairs serve a noble purpose? By breathing through the nose, you are working with your body's anatomy.

The Exhale

Breathe in through your nose, hold, and then breathe out through your mouth. Notice, are you exhaling for at least as long as you are inhaling? Why does that matter? Our exhale is a mini-detox. We are releasing what remains of the "used" oxygen.

Think about the inhale as nourishing each cell in your body with oxygen, and the exhale removing the stale air. The inhale enjoying fresh oxygen. The exhale making room for that next inhale.

Practice a full exhale right now and notice how you feel. Count as you are breathing in, and then count as you are breathing out. Aim to have the exhale be as long or longer than the inhale. Try it now.

Tactical Cue

Sit up straight or lie on your back. Place one hand on your chest and one on your upper abdomen (above the belly button and below the ribs). Aim to have the hand on your upper abdomen rise and fall as you breathe.

Fairy Wings

Picture the shape of your lungs. Notice how they are roughly the same shape as fairy wings? Picture yourself breathing in love all the way down to the tips of your fairy wings. As you breathe out, picture that you are flapping your fairy wings. Enjoy your love-powered breath as you fly in the direction of your true north.

Bursts

Sit up straight. Breathe in and out of your nose in short equal bursts. There are many variations of this particular breath, so you can experiment to see what feels right for you. I like to do it for 10 – 15 seconds, followed by a nice steady breath, and then repeat for a second round.

Nourishing our Cells with Hydration

When I was a Peace Corps Volunteer, the US Government provided us training before sending us to live in remote villages for two years. One aspect of our training was hydration. As you are reading this Guidebook, if you are lucky enough to have easy access to safe drinking water, that is a reason to celebrate. Truly.

Let's start from a place of gratitude as we begin to think about the ways we can nourish our bodies with water. Things like climate, your activity level, and your size will all play a role in how much you need to drink. Which means it will vary. It does become easier to work with your body to find that right balance once staying hydrated is part of your conscious decision making.

The next thing I'd like to cover is the color of your output. I didn't want to totally shock you by moving straight in with this topic, but now that you are ready, let's talk about the color of your urine. As a general gauge, if it is light yellow, you are likely in that hydration sweet spot. If it is water-clear, you may be drinking too much water. If it starts moving into medium yellow, that's a sign that you are likely not drinking enough water. While we are talking about urine, be aware that there are some supplements that can temporarily change the color of your urine. And eating beets can change the color also! If you are in doubt, consult your healthcare professional.

Hydration is an important component in our body's (and our brain's) healthy function. There is a lot of science to back up the importance of staying hydrated. Our bodies need water to function properly. Think about your blood pumping through your body transporting nutrients and oxygen to all the cells. Or about the saliva that begins your digestion process. Or about the waste products that we remove when we urinate. Or about your sweat that regulates your body temperature. From a how-we-look perspective, when we get dehydrated, our skin looks less elastic and youthful.

Another bonus reason to stay hydrated is that when you exercise, being hydrated allows you to maximize your power and endurance, and it reduces fatigue. Plus, if you are a Mom or an Auntie or a role model with little eyes watching you, staying hydrated models healthy water drinking habits. Hopefully, you've found your motivation, now let's talk about making water-drinking fun!

Two and a half tips for getting in your H_2O every day
H_2O Tip One

Bring a big glass or water bottle of water with you up to bed and leave it bedside. In the morning, start your day by drinking it. How much water will you be starting your day with? You can experiment with the amount to figure out what feels right for your body. A great starting place is 10-12 ounces of water.

H_2O Tip Two

The next one and a half tips have to do with jazzing up your water. If sipping water throughout the day isn't coming easily for you, then you may want to try creating a water bar. The water bar consists of fun and healthy water add-ins that make drinking water more fun. What are some add-in examples? A wedge of lemon, a sprig of mint, frozen organic blueberries. Can you think of other fun things you could add to your water bar?

Here are a few more ideas... low glycemic fruit such as lime or raspberries, organic herbs such as basil, or a slice of cut cucumber. Do any of those sound appealing to you? Which one or two might you be willing to give a try this week? What day are you thinking about doing it? Can you visualize yourself enjoying your tasty refreshing water? Can you visualize setting up your water bar fixings on a cutting board on your counter? Can you visualize storing the prepared fixings in the fridge?

H_20 Tip Two and a half

The other half tip is to take the water bar to a bit zestier level. If you occasionally seek out the after dinner drink, you may want to notice, is it the effects of the alcohol you are seeking out, or might it be the ritual you have created around that evening drink? How do you DO your after dinner drink? Is it a time of day you have carved out to relax? Do you breath more deeply? Do you allow yourself to have a quiet moment as you take the first sip? Notice how you DO that drink.

Think about how to create a water-based ritual with all those same elements. For example, if you have a ritual that includes a glass of wine, instead try a glass or two of Pellegrino in a wine glass with frozen blueberries. Even though on the surface the almost $2 for a pint of Pellegrino may seem high, when you compare it to the cost of a glass of your favorite wine or spirit you may be saving yourself money. (In addition to getting your hydration on.) If a quiet warm drink is what you seek... perhaps see if hot water with lemon can quench your thirst and your ritual. Here's to your hydration!!!

Nourishing our Cells with Flowing Energy

The flow of energy is talked about matter-of-factly in so many cultures. I believe one day in our lifetimes, it will become more common to measure our energy body and with those feedback devices of the future, energy hygiene will likely become much more common practice. However for now, I recognize that this suggestion may be bumping against the edge of comfort. Therefore I offer this as a consideration and if it resonates with you, great. And if not, that's ok too. It's food for thought.

As you are moving throughout your day, notice if you are holding tension in your body. Notice if you are clenching your muscles or holding your breath. Consider what that might mean if we do in fact have energy currents trying to run through our bodies and nourish our cells. If you picture the energy as water (something tangible and therefore easier to visualize), imagine what happens when water gets blocked, pooled up, stagnant and stale. Can you visualize the difference between stale and flowing water? Which one seems full of vigor and vitality? Which would you rather have running through you?

If you are still with me and still comfortable with the topic, do a self-check, and notice where in your body you may be blocking your flow. Once you identify a spot, see if you can breathe with your attention focused on that area and loosen up that tension or block. Why not try it right now.

If you tried it, how did it feel?

Fuel Drop Two: Nourishing Our Hearts

One of our human needs is for connection. When we don't consciously seek out ways to fill ourselves up with positive connection, we sometimes find ourselves turning to unhealthy approaches to connection, like eating or other short-term faux connection. Nourishing our hearts and fueling up with healthy connection does not require a romantic partner. Even if you do have a romantic partner that lights up your world, nourishing our hearts begins with ourselves.

There are many different approaches for filling our need for nourishing our hearts. The key is that you CONSCIOUSLY choose how you fuel up with connection. Below are some examples of ways we can fuel ourselves with love and connection.

Volunteering

One amazingly fulfilling way to enhance our own lives and at the same time add value to the lives of those around us is to connect by volunteering some of our time. Time is a very precious resource, so it may be that you only have a sparse amount of time that you are able to budget for volunteering. That's ok. Take a look at your time budget and decide an amount of time that you can comfortable allocate without going past your exhaustion point and without going past your resentment point. Once you determine what that time budget is, commit to giving your focused and heartfelt attention while you volunteer, however large or small that timeslot may be.

Connect with yourself

A powerful way to meet our human need for love and connection is to love and connect with ourselves. We can do this by accepting ourselves as we are. We thrive best when we see, accept, and love all of the many **hues of our human-ness**.

Authentic connection with loved ones

How do we nourish our hearts with authentic connection? When we see, accept, and appreciate ourselves as we are **and** our loved ones as they are, we cultivate authentic connection. Our capacity to accept other people is often related to how well we embrace our own selves, which is why connection with self is part of the equation.

Religious and/or Spiritual Practices

If you have a religious or spiritual practice that resonates with you and fuels you, that can be another beautiful way to connect and to nourish your heart.

So far we've talked about four examples of how we can fuel up on loving connection. What some other ways of nourishing your heart that come to mind?

Creativity

How about expressing yourself creatively? What would that look like for you? Creativity is not limited to the traditional arts. It could be in the way you cut your lemon wedge for your water bar. You can be creative with your spreadsheets.

The nourishment comes in expressing yourself. How do you currently express yourself creatively? In what other ways might you want to express yourself creatively?

<u>Forgiveness</u>

When we carry around anger or resentment, we are impeding our maximum potential for nourishing our hearts. When we forgive, we lessen the burden on our own wellness. It's not always easy to do, and it's not always our first human reaction. If you find that you keep coming back to a certain person or a certain event and playing it over and over again, that may be a sign that you are holding yourself back from your maximum wellness.

One thing you may want to consider is allowing yourself whatever natural reaction you have, even if it is not forgiveness. Then notice your reaction and recognize if it becomes persistent or debilitating. Start asking yourself questions. Get curious with yourself. Start to paint the picture of your life six months from now, or two years from now, if you choose to set yourself free.

<u>Fun</u>

One last fun way to nourish our hearts... fun! Whatever your definition of fun is... whether it's laughter, or hiking in nature, dancing in the moonlight, writing, playing music, cooking, hanging out with friends... there are tons of vitality-boosting ways to have fun and in the process nourish our hearts.

IMPORTANT ASSIGNMENT

Here's your assignment for fuel drop two: try to do something fun this week. Even if you are totally busy and all you can carve out is a 15-minute block of time. Do it!

Fuel Drop Three: Rest and Rejuvenation

Balancing all of the important pieces of our lives can be such a challenge for so many of us, which makes getting a full night sleep almost burdensome. It's tricky because we don't know how long we'll have in these human vehicles to experience all the joy life has to offer; and yet, our human vehicles are our mode for getting around for however long we are here. The kinder we are to our bodies, the more vigor and vitality we have to enjoy the time we are here.

Plus, getting enough sleep can **improve cognitive function** and lack of sleep can be a cause for food cravings. Which would you rather experience?

Want to support your body in getting an optimal amount of sleep? Create a bedtime ritual. A good starting point for creating your ritual is to calculate the target time to be in bed. Think about what time you need to wake up in the morning and then back up what time you would need to go to go sleep in order to wake up rested. Then factor in how long it usually takes to fall asleep and that gives you your target time to be in bed. If seeing that time in writing evokes a feeling of pressure then *yeah, you just uncovered a wellness blocker.*

I know, believe me I know, when you really look at your **time budget**, it usually leads to an exercise in how you want to prioritize. As challenging as it is to make quality decisions about what you want to say no to, it's important to make those conscious choices rather than not look at it and inadvertently sacrifice your higher priorities.

Think about what activities you do right before bed. One will be to get your water ready and placed bedside for your morning hydration. What are other activities? What else do you do as you prepare for bed? Once you list everything out, start to visualize the order that you do these things. Is it the same each night? Now figure out how long it will take you to do these activities. That gives you your target start time for your bedtime ritual.

When you make the tiny shift in your language and you start thinking about these activities as a ritual, you are signaling to your body that you are preparing for sleep, which can set you up for a more restful night sleep. The more clearly we communicate with our bodies, the more likely we are to be in harmony with ourselves and deepen our wellness.

Other restful-night-sleep-promoting techniques to consider include:

- If your schedule allows for it, aim to get into a pattern for going to sleep at approximately the same time each night.
- If you drink caffeine - don't drink it after a certain time. You can experiment with your own body for what that optimal time is. Is it noon? Earlier than that? Later than that?

- For our hydration, consider slowing down or stopping your water intake a couple of hours before bed so you can avoid the sleep interruption of having a full bladder.
- Consider turning off your cell phone about an hour before going to bed.
- Consider staying off electronics, including TV and computer for about an hour before going to bed a few nights a week.
- If your head is still full of thoughts that are keeping you awake, try taking a nice big breath with the goal of clearing your mind and preparing it for a restful and replenishing night sleep. You may even find that the solution for whatever it is you are mulling over becomes more apparent when you wake up refreshed and rejuvenated.

Rejuvenation

In addition to sleeping, do you think there are other ways you can rejuvenate? It may not be realistic to build in enough time for a full night's sleep plus add additional time for rejuvenation at this time, but let's briefly touch on it so we can plant an aspirational seed of things to come.

It could be something simple like take a hot bath with music playing or standing barefoot on the ground outside in the summertime for five minutes. Take a couple of minutes right now to either think about or write down some of the activities that leave you feeling rejuvenated.

What's the item on the list that takes the least time? Do you think it will be possible to build time into your schedule to do it in the next week? If it's not possible right now, can you look out a month and budget a little bit of time for rejuvenation? What is your favorite thing on your rejuvenation list? Does just thinking about it bring a smile to your face? Sometimes rejuvenation is simply a matter of focusing on the thing that make us smile.

Fuel Drop Review

Now that we've talked in more detail about all three of our Human Vehicle Basics fuel drops, let's review them:

Fuel Drop One: Nourishing our Cells
Fuel Drop Two: Nourishing our Hearts
Fuel Drop Three: Rest and Rejuvenation

Coming up next, we'll be talking about our Internal Terrain, which includes food sensitivities and our hormones, but first, let's review the key take-aways from this chapter.

Key Take-aways
Human Vehicle Basics

Our bodies are fueled on much more than just the food we eat. In this chapter, we focused on the foundational fuel for our human vehicles.

Fuel Drop One: Nourishing our Cells
- I appreciate that my body breathes whether or not I am focusing on my breath, thank you body
- I aim to remember to take deep, cell-nourishing breaths every day
- Being hydrated is awesome

Fuel Drop Two: Nourishing our Hearts
- I choose to approach my human need for connection by fueling myself with positive connection
- I aim to make conscious choices for how I nourish my heart

Fuel Drop Three: Rest and Rejuvenation
- I will consider creating a bedtime ritual
- I will aim to budget some time for rejuvenation

Chapter Eight
Internal Terrain

In this chapter, we'll be talking about our Internal Terrain and the things we can do to keep our insides happy. The three fuel drops are:

Fuel Drop One: Food Sensitivities
Fuel Drop Two: Happy Belly
Fuel Drop Three: Hormones

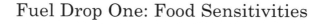

Fuel Drop One: Food Sensitivities

Let's start with Food Sensitivities because, as you might imagine, your belly is likely not as happy as it could be if you are eating foods your body doesn't tolerate well. If you have an extreme and obvious food allergy or an extreme and obvious food sensitivity, it's likely that you already know about it; and if it's uncomfortable enough, you likely steer clear of it. If it's not terribly uncomfortable, it probably depends on how tasty it is as to whether or not you completely avoid it or occasionally eat it. Either way, it's likely that you know about it. However, what if it's not such an obvious reaction?

When the reaction isn't extreme and it isn't immediate, we don't always associate it with the specific food that may have caused it. Our human vehicles are so complex; there are so many interactions happening in our bodies, it's really quite amazing.

111

The challenge in navigating that complexity is that as advanced as our sciences are in certain respects, we are not yet able to measure the impact of every food and every ingredient we consume because there are so many variables.

When we focus on all of the chemical, biological, and electrical interactions going on in our bodies, it can become daunting. Let's remind ourselves that yes, our human vehicles are complex, but our inner wisdom has a knowing that will support us. With a mind-set of leveraging whatever good science is available, AND ALSO trusting our inner wisdom let's talk more about food sensitivities.

Food sensitivities can show up in many forms. Some common symptoms of food sensitivities are bloating, hives, migraines, fogginess, and sluggishness. It's tricky because you can experience those symptoms as a result of food sensitivities or something other than food. It gets even more complicated, but don't worry, we'll also talk about solutions... it gets more complicated because response times can vary. Sometimes they are immediate, and sometimes they are delayed by a couple of hours or by a couple of days.

When we fuel our bodies with foods that we have sensitivities to, we are fueling ourselves, but at the same time, we are also creating more work for our bodies to do. As amazing as our bodies are, they have to make some choices as to where to apply the resources. If we introduce a food that our body doesn't tolerate well, our body will apply some of its resources to respond to the offending food.

When we become more aware of how our bodies are reacting, we are able to make more informed decisions about what fuels our bodies well.

Food Sensitivities Action Plan
Step 1: Notice

Start paying attention to how you feel. Check in with yourself regularly. When you are choosing between a meal with less ingredients or more ingredients, if you would enjoy them both, consider opting for the one with less ingredients.

Step 2: Conscious Decision Making and Information Gathering

Conscious decision making is not about making new food rules, it's about making informed decisions. It's helpful to understand the consequences of the choices we are making rather than walk around feeling off and not knowing why.

To give you an example, I have a food sensitivity to tomatoes and to yeast. Before I zeroed in on those specific foods I did notice that every time I ate pizza, I felt super tired and bloated. What did I do after I noticed that every time I ate pizza I didn't have the energy to do the things that fuel me and bring me the most happiness? At first what I did was I decided I was only going to eat pizza on Friday nights, which is a time in my schedule that it's usually ok for me to get tired and crash on the couch to watch a movie or just simply go to bed extra early. This is what I mean by conscious decision-making.

Interestingly enough, eventually, it wasn't worth it to me. Even though I don't have any personal rules that say I can't eat pizza, I choose not to because I have experienced the consequences of that choice enough to know that for my body, the pros of eating a delicious slice of pizza do not outweigh the cons.

Step 3: Start a food sensitivity journal or document

Every time you notice you aren't feeling at the top of your game, whether you're bloated, you feel foggy, you notice extra mucus, you get a migraine ... even if you don't think it's food related, just jot it down. When you jot down the symptoms, also try to remember what you've recently eaten and when. If you happen to remember, include in the entry what you just ate, what you ate a couple of hours ago, what you ate within the last 24 hours, and within the last 48 hours. As you collect this information slowly, over time, you may notice a pattern.

Here are a few examples to get your mind warmed up and ready to be on the lookout for your patterns. Just keep in mind, this is just a few of many possibilities.

- Maybe every time you eat a certain dish, you feel bloated 15 minutes later
- Or maybe every time you eat a certain dish, an hour later you are craving a certain food
- Or every time you eat a certain food, the next morning your hands are a little bit swollen
- Or you feel hung-over even though you didn't drink alcohol
- Or every time you eat a certain food or a certain dish, you get a runny nose two days later

These are just some of the many patterns you can be on the lookout for. When you do notice a pattern, you can then move on to step 4 to explore further. We can learn a lot of information if we pay attention and jot down notes here and there.

Step number 4: Further Exploration

If you suspect a food sensitivity, I recommend that you eliminate that food for 21 days and then reintroduce it at the end of the 21 days and observe how your body responds to the food. Why 21 days? The first place I was exposed to the concept of a 21-day elimination period was twenty years ago when I read Dr. Berger's *Immune Power Diet* book. In it, he shared his own research as to why he thought 21 days was the right amount of time based on his experience as a physician working with his many patients. Since then, in addition to using it as a tool myself, there have been many programs that use that same 21-day formula with success. It's a powerful tool and if it resonates with you, I highly recommend it.

Once you've eliminated a food item for 21 days when you reintroduce it, usually the response becomes more obvious and therefore easier to observe. The observable response gives you the information to make an informed decision about eating that particular food.

Is going for 21 days without a food item that you enjoy challenging? It definitely can be, but I don't recommend willful ignorance. If you suspect a food sensitivity, it's better to investigate. If you have a specific food item that you can't imagine going without for 21 days, you might want to take a deeper look at that relationship. We all have foods we love, but 'enjoying' and 'being dependent upon' are two different things. As always, be kind to yourself as you explore what's right for you and your body.

Common Food Sensitivities

The next thing we are going to talk about is common food sensitivities that you can be on the lookout for. If you are interested in accelerating the process of finding your food sensitivities you can eliminate foods that commonly cause food sensitivities and then slowly reintroduce them, one food at a time. When I say one food at a time, that means one new food every three days.

If you are thinking about eliminating multiple food items at one time, the one heads up I'll give you is that eliminating multiple food items at one time has some pros and some cons. It does give you the opportunity to gather data faster. But it also means being very patient as you reintroduce foods one at a time no faster than one every three days. Don't underestimate that time because when you tack three days onto the end of a 21-day elimination period, you have more than 21 days, so choose wisely.

What are those common foods? I'll share **three** lists with you. One is from the CDC. (The CDC is short for United States Center for Disease Control and Prevention, which is a national public health institute.) The second is Dr. Stuart Berger's sinister seven, and I'll explain to you why I've included that list. The third is my personal Top Foods to Watch list

CDC List

Let's start with the CDC list. In 2008 the CDC published a public paper that stated that eight types of food account for over 90% of allergic reactions among minors in the United States. The eight foods they named were:

1. Milk
2. Eggs
3. Peanuts
4. Tree nuts
5. Fish
6. Shellfish
7. Soy
8. Wheat

Dr. Berger's List

Dr. Berger's list includes some of the same items that are on the CDC list. The reason I am also including Dr. Berger's list of common food sensitivities is for three reasons. One, the CDC research studied people under eighteen. Secondly, the CDC list is food allergies and typically when you have an allergy, you already know about it. The other important reason I am including Dr. Berger's list is because the CDC's list does not include sugar or corn and there are many well-researched resources that suggest many people have reactions to those foods.

The items in common with the CDC list are: Milk, Eggs, Soy, and Wheat. In addition, his list includes: Corn, Yeast, and Cane Sugar

Simona's Top Foods to Watch List

My list starts with the "sinister seven" from Dr. Berger's list. It also includes shellfish from the CDC list. Plus, my list adds nightshades and MSG.

What are nightshades? 'Nightshades' is the term used for a group of plants that includes tomatoes, eggplant, peppers, and white potatoes (but not sweet potatoes), and paprika. For those that have food sensitivities to nightshades, one of the common ways that sensitivity shows up is with inflammation, and inflammation does not make for a healthy internal terrain. MSG is on the list because of its long list of common adverse reactions.

These are not in order of importance because the one that is most important is whichever one you are sensitive to.
1. Milk
2. Eggs
3. Soy
4. Wheat
5. Corn
6. Yeast
7. Cane Sugar
8. Shellfish
9. Nightshades
10. MSG

Wrapping up Fuel Drop One

During fuel drop one we talked about paying attention to how you feel and jotting down some notes so that over time you can notice if there are any patterns that may suggest a correlation between what you ate and how you felt. We also talked about eliminating any suspicious food for 21 days and then observing how you feel when you reintroduce it. And, we talked about making informed choices. Here's wishing you that everything you eat yields health and harmony within!

Fuel Drop Two: Happy Belly

A happy belly, or really a happy digestive tract, is one that can assimilate the nutrients we offer our bodies and eliminate the rest. We've already practiced a couple tools on our path to having a happy belly. Let's review those first as we kick off fuel drop two.

Tools for a Happy Belly

One tool is to chew. During our *How We Eat Matters* chapter, one of our fuel drops was Presentness In Our Meals and one of the techniques we talked about was chewing. When we are present in our meals, we are also supporting our healthy internal terrain. Chewing is the start of the mechanical and chemical process of digestion.

Chewing
Why is chewing a tool for a happy digestive tract?
- Chewing breaks your food down from the bite you put into your mouth into smaller particles that can be more easily digested.

119

- As we chew, we are sending signals to the rest of our digestive tract to get prepared for digestion.

- Saliva contains digestive enzymes, so the longer you chew, the more time the enzymes have to start breaking down the food you are eating.

We may not remember to chew thoroughly at every single meal, or even every single day, but now that you know it is important, you may find that you do chew more some of the time. When you chew more, aim to notice how you are feeling an hour later or a day later. Notice your energy level. Chewing a little more can really make a difference.

The more often you intentionally chew more, the more you'll build the habit. Small tweaks can take us very far along our path of vibrant wellness. Do you think you can commit to every once in a while, when you think of it, chewing more when you eat?

The Digestion Zone

The other tool that you already have in your tool-belt for a happy belly is the first Z in A-W-E-Z-Z, the digestion zone. In the *5 Daily Basics* chapter, we talked about allowing time for our bodies to convert the food we already ate into fuel. What that means is to be mindful of how much time you wait between snacks and meals. When we honor the digestion zone, we give the food time to travel through the digestive tract to be chemically broken down and converted into energy.

A key benefit of honoring the digestion zone is more energy. And, it doesn't take any time out of our busy day to do it! To learn the simple steps for how to calculate the time between meals, check out the appendix of your Guidebook or visit our website FueltheBodyWell.com. You can also find a free Digestion Zone timer app in the iTunes store.

Can you visualize when you are going to have your next opportunity to honor the digestion zone? When is that going to be? Today? Tomorrow? The reason we take the time to visualize it is because when you can picture yourself doing it, you are setting yourself up for greater success on your wellness path.

The ecosystem in our gut

We are still talking about our happy bellies, but we are about to shift our discussion to bacteria in our guts, so I wanted to give you a moment to shift your focus so you are ready. Ready?

There is a lot going on in our guts. It's an entire ecosystem filled with living organisms. There's scientific agreement that there are an enormous amount of bacteria in our guts and there is also agreement that some of these bacteria can be considered "good" or beneficial and some can be considered "bad" or harmful. However when it comes to the question of how to feed those living organisms in our gut for optimal wellness, the messages are mixed.

When messages are mixed, I like to look at the situation from a few angles. I look at the research, at the long timeline of human history (vs. looking at an immediate fad), at the experience of the experts in the field that came before me, and at first-hand personal experience. That information is a helpful starting point and then from there, armed with baseline information, we can pay attention to what works for our own bodies. Are you up for noticing what works for your own body?

Let's start with that baseline information so you have a starting point. In addition to nourishing our bodies with fueling food choices, optimal gut wellness includes feeding the beneficial bacteria and not feeding the harmful bacteria. Two of the most common recommendations for what to eat and what not to eat for gut health are:
1. Eating fermented foods like sauerkraut or kimchi
2. Eating less sugar

Why sauerkraut?

The fermentation process produces probiotics that replenish and support the beneficial bacteria in your gut. An added bonus is that sauerkraut is a great tool in our tool belt for combating food cravings. If you can't stand sauerkraut or kimchi, you may want to consider taking a probiotic. You can talk to your nutritionally informed healthcare provider for a recommendation of which might be best for you.

Why the recommendation to eat less sugar?

Sugar feeds the harmful bacteria. It's interesting to think about sugar on a human-history timeline to realize that for most of our existence as human beings, lack of food was much more of a concern than over-filling our guts. As a species, we gravitate towards sweet, delicious food like fresh, local, in season fruit. However, when you speed up the timeline of human history you'll see sugar goes from something we ate when we found fruit seasonally, to something that was cultivated but the price was so high that only a few could afford it, to industrial improvements in the middle of eighteenth century that led to lower cost and increased demand.

According to physiologist and nutritionist John Yudkin in his book *Pure, White, and Deadly* world sugar production grew from 3.8 million metric tons in 1880 to 101 million metric tons in 1980. According to the USDA (the United States Department of Agriculture), sugar production for the 2013/2014 fiscal year was 175.7 million metric tons.

What does this brief history of sugar have to do with our happy bellies? It's a reminder that eating the amount of sugar we eat today is a relatively new human trend, and as our ability to measure the impact of that change improves, we are learning that increasing our sugar consumption that dramatically has an impact to our overall wellness.

I am not suggesting that you replace sugar with chemical substitutes. What I am suggesting is simply being aware of when you are eating sugar and, when possible, to consider reducing your sugar consumption without making extreme food rules that leave you feeling deprived and ready to rebel against yourself.

What else can we do to support our happy bellies?

As we nurture and nourish our bodies in a way that encourages assimilation of nutrients as well as elimination of the by-products that our bodies do not need, we are supporting our happy bellies. We've already talked about some terrific ways we can nurture and nourish our bodies, including being mindful of our negative stress and eating foods that are fueling. Another tool is movement, which we'll be talking about in chapter eleven. If you are looking for even more tools for supporting our happy bellies, let's talk enzymes.

Ann Wigmore, a twentieth century naturopath and homeopath, the original founder of the Hippocrates Health Institute in Boston, and the founder of the Ann Wigmore Natural Health Institute in Puerto Rico, emphasized the importance of supporting a balanced internal environment in the gut through eating enzyme-rich foods as well as being mindful of avoiding foods that disrupt the balance in the gut.

She goes into details about the prominent enzymes and their role in digestion in her teachings, but what I'd like to talk about with you here is a visual she gave that I still use as a tool for focusing my thoughts towards choosing gut-loving options a lot of the time. When we think about our enzymes like a bank account it simplifies our choices. We can make choices to "deposit" or add to our enzyme account, such as eating nourishing foods. And we can make choices that "withdraw" from our enzyme account such as eating processed, chemicalized foods. The goal is to keep our enzyme bank net positive.

What do you think of that image? Does it motivate you to want to keep a positive balance? As we wrap up this fuel drop, let's think about one small action we can take today that adds to the happiness of our bellies.

Fuel Drop Three: Hormones

The very first thing I'd like to say on the topic of hormones is that our female bodies are amazing. We are so complex, so special, and so very wonderful. Yes, our hormones can be challenging to figure out. It can occasionally be so frustrating that our bodies are different from week to week as we move through various stages in our cycle, and even different from life stage to life stage. But we have a choice . . . we can either think about this complexity as a burden or as the gift that is. Our amazingness is so vast but unfortunately, our cultural conditioning does not always reinforce or remind us of that.

Personally, I can thank my shifting hormones because they are great teachers. When my hormones shift, I hold on to these fuel drops and they allow me to continue to live my well life. When I say your wellness path can become effortless, I mean it in two very important ways. I mean that by practicing these fuel drops, you may find that as you make small adjustments to your lifestyle that it becomes increasingly more intuitive to make choices that fuel your vibrant wellness. I also mean that by practicing these fuel drops, you may develop that reflexive muscle memory that reminds you to reach out for your fuel drops when you need them.

Even though my hormone shifts can be like a rough sea, by reaching out for the fuel drops, I can often quickly rebalance and return to quieter seas. That's important because the fact of the matter is, our hormones will continue to shift. They shift throughout our moon cycles and throughout our lifetimes. They shift from girlhood to young womanhood during puberty and they shift again starting generally between age 35 and 40 towards wise womanhood. The medical term for the shift towards wise womanhood is perimenopause, but unfortunately there is too much talk about it as if it were a disease or condition rather than being what it is, which is a beautiful transition. This transition connects us to an even deeper and wiser feminine power and beauty within ourselves.

It's not a question of if our bodies are shifting;
it's a matter of how we navigate those shifts.

Navigating our hormone shifts

Fortunately, lifestyle tweaks can go a long way in alleviating many of the common symptoms associated with out-of-balance hormones. It is my perspective that the frustration of our shifting hormones could be partially mitigated if we had better tools and information to navigate what we are experiencing. One thing that helps me to stay in appreciation and gratitude of the complexity rather than focus on the frustration of navigating the seemingly constant changes is when I compare it to the navigation tools for ancient travel vs. modern day travel. In ancient times, they had some hand drawn maps based on the people's experiences that came before them. However today, we can travel the world with GPS-precision. With information, what was once complex becomes common.

With that in mind, although our society's current understanding of a woman's hormones is unfortunately not yet to the level of the navigation tools we have for modern day travel, let's take a look at the maps we do have.

Let's dive in by starting with a definition. Of all of the definitions and descriptions I have read, my favorite explanation of hormones comes from Donna Eden. She says in her *Energy Medicine for Women* book "If you think of each cell in your body as a theater with a thousand stages, hormones raise and lower the curtains".

When you think about it as raising and lowering the curtains, it's easier to visualize that each hormone has a job to do. If you are interested in the science and interplay between the various hormones, a great resource is Dr. Sara Gottfried's book, *The Hormone Cure*.

Here's a quick summary of some terms that commonly come up when the topic of hormones is being discussed.

- There are our Adrenal Glands, which are small glands, which happen to be located on top of each kidney. They are most known for producing cortisol
- Cortisol is your main stress hormone
- There's Thyroid, which affects your metabolism
- And our primary reproductive organs: the ovaries, which produce Estrogen and Progesterone

There are many different possibilities and combinations of possibilities for why our bodies are not always responding the way we expect them to, which is why it's really helpful when we can collaborate with our own inner wisdom on our wellness path.

If your head is starting to spin right about now, and you'd just like to have a solution, I have a great tool for you. It's not a magic bullet, but I have found it makes a huge difference for many women. It's the 3-minute Routine we learned about in the *5 Daily Basics* chapter. You can find the details about how to do the routine in the appendix of you Guidebook.

The reason why the 3-minute Routine is my first-line tool is because stress can really put a wrench in the works. Hormones will shift with or without negative stress in our bodies, but in the absence of negative stress, when our bodies are healthy they often find their way back to balance. The less negative stress we have, the better we are able to ride the wave of those shifts with a little more understanding.

That's not always the case, but it's the case often enough that it merits our attention. When we experience stress, our loving bodies go into protection mode. They look out for our well-being. When our bodies are working to save us, they are directing most resources towards surviving the immediate threat.

With the visual that our hormones are raising and lowering the curtains in the theater of our cells, you can now visualize that they are super busy raising and lowering curtains all over the body navigating what is needed based on the stress signal we sent out. By doing the 3-minute Routine, we are communicating with our bodies and letting them know that we are experiencing modern stress and that we are not in a life-threatening situation. Clear communication takes you a long way on your wellness path.

Fuel Drop Review

Now that we've talked in more detail about all three of our fuel drops, let's review them:

Fuel Drop One: Food Sensitivities
Fuel Drop Two: Happy Belly
Fuel Drop Three: Hormones

Here's wishing you a happy and healthy internal terrain! In the next chapter we'll be talking about what foods fuel YOUR body well.

Key Take-aways
Internal Terrain

Fuel Drop One: Food Sensitivities

- I am confident that I can fuel and operate my human vehicle with grace
- I pay attention to how I feel after eating and jot down notes so that over time I can notice if there are any patterns
- As I patiently become more aware of how my body is reacting to the foods I eat, I am able to make more informed decisions about what fuels MY body well

Fuel Drop Two: Happy Belly

- I aim to nurture and nourish my body in a way that encourages assimilation of the nutrients (and elimination of the by-products)
- Some of the ways I can nurture and nourish my body include: being mindful of negative stress, eating foods that are fueling, and movement

Fuel Drop Three: Hormones

- There are so many gifts that are inherent in residing in my fascinating and wonderful female body
- I will aim to reach out for my favorite fuel drops to support me in navigating hormone shifts
- I will aim to learn the 3-minute Routine

Chapter Nine
Nourishing Foods

In this chapter we'll be talking about how we can leverage food to create extraordinary energy and vitality. You'll be learning tools for choosing what to eat to fuel YOUR body well without having to wonder if you should be following the food-trend du jour. Before we dive into the fuel drops, let's do a fun exercise so we can set the stage for getting the maximum benefit.

Fuel Flower Exercise

To get started, I have a question for you.... did you learn the food pyramid when you were growing up? I ask because if you did, that means at a very impressionable age, you learned a one-size fits all eating solution. You also learned an exclusively food-focused methodology. The fuel flower reminds us that our bodies are individual, and while we are certainly similar to other people, we are each unique. Therefore, what fuels each of our bodies well is also similar and yet unique. Our fuel flowers also remind us that food is only part of the way we fuel our bodies well.

This is a three-step exercise and will probably take you two or three minutes to do unless you want to take it to the next level and decide to draw a beautiful flower so you can hang it up... and if you are inspired to do that, go for it!

Fuel Flower Step 1

Create a list of things that fuel your body well.

Here are a few to get your ideas flowing:

- Smiles
- Laughter
- Gratitude
- A positive relationship with yourself
- *Awesome* cell nourishing breaths

Fuel Flower Step 2

Draw a flower with as many petals as you have fuels. You may also want to add a few extra petals in case you think of something more later. Then, fill in the petals with your words

Fuel Flower Step 3

Once you've filled in the words, look at your Fuel Flower and allow your eyes to soak in the message. Our fuel flowers can remind us that us of our own personal recipe for fueling ourselves for a Vibrant and Well life.

Nourishing Foods Fuel Drops

With our fuel flowers in-hand, let's dive in to the three Fuel Drops:

Fuel Drop One: Food As Fuel
Fuel Drop Two: Macro and Micro Nutrients
Fuel Drop Three: What Foods Fuel YOUR Body Well

Fuel Drop One: Food As Fuel

When we start to think about food as fuel for our beautiful human vehicles, our food choices can become a little clearer. Does that mean that everything we choose to eat will be nourishing? Probably not. Most likely, even with our growing awareness of what fuels our bodies well, and even with our deepening connection with our inner wisdom, we may still occasionally use food for things it is not designed to fuel.

That's ok. It's human of us. The cool thing is that as we stay curious, observant, and radically honest with ourselves about the choices we are making, we start to make more fueling choices, more of the time. If we were to put our food choices through the filter of 'food as fuel', does it make it easier to discern which foods may be more nourishing? Does it help to picture the food converting into a clean and steady source of energy? Energy that you can use to do the things that you NEED to do, plus have plenty of energy to also do the things you WANT to do. We are not talking about the kind of energy that borrows from tomorrow, but truly fueling in the now; having ABUNDANT ENERGY day-after-day. Does that sound good?

Let's take a moment right now to check in and notice if there is any noise getting in the way of clear communication with our inner wisdom. When I asked you if that sounded good, what did you think? Did you like the idea of more energy? Did you think it sounded feasible? Did you have multiple thoughts about the question… and were some of them in conflict?

It's ok if you have conflicting thoughts. The important thing is to be aware of what thoughts are running in the foreground as well as the background. When we notice all of our thoughts, even the ones that are conflicting with one another, we have more information to navigate in the direction we choose.

I am going to ask you one more time.... when I asked you if that sounds good, what do you think? Now that we've had a moment to check in with ourselves and clean out some potential static, let's talk more about Food As Fuel.

Fuel Filter Question

If I ask you if an ice cream sundae seems like it would be nourishing, what would you say?

Notice the question, the question we are talking about at the moment is not 'do I want to eat this'. It is not 'am I going to choose to eat this whether or not it is nourishing'. The question is 'will this nourish me'? Or said another way, will this give me the fuel I need to do all the things I NEED to do, plus have plenty of energy to do the things I WANT to do.

How about a soda?

What about corn on the cob?

When we talk about corn on the cob we are getting into what fuels YOUR body well because corn on the cob will be fueling for some bodies but not for every body.

Asking yourself the right question as you are choosing what to eat is a simple, yet powerful tool. Keep in mind, just because you ask the question, doesn't mean you have to abide by the answer. It's just information so you can make a conscious choice.

My Fuel Filter question is 'will this fuel my body well'. Does that question resonate with you? If so, give it a try at your next meal. If not, write your own now. What is your fuel filter question going to be?

Food Philosophy

People often ask me what my food philosophy is. Am I a vegan? Do I follow paleo? Low fat? High fat? Low carb? High carb? During fuel drop three, we will talk about why so many different food philosophies can report success stories. Right now, I'd like to share my food philosophy because it has everything to do with fuel drop one.

What is my food philosophy? It's asking the question: 'Will this fuel my body well?'. With that information I make conscious and informed choices about what I eat. Does that mean that what I eat is boring? No way. Fueling can co-exist with fun and delicious. Does that mean I always eat to fuel my body well? Not always, and that's ok. What it does mean is that I am making fueling choices for myself a lot of the time.

It also means, when I choose to eat something for other reasons I am clear and aware of those choices. Why is that helpful? For one, it means I do it without guilt; and guilt is not

135

awesome for your wellness. Plus, if my body is trying to communicate with me, I will be more likely to hear the message. It also means that I can consciously notice how I feel later and use it as a data point for future decision-making.

By asking ourselves the question, we are awakening our awareness of cause and effect. Fueling the body well is not about restricting. It's about lovingly nourishing ourselves. It's about getting to experience what life feels like when we make fueling decisions more of the time. I'd like to encourage you to try out your fuel filter question. What do you think? Is that something you'd be willing to try?

Whether or not you are going to try it out this week, or some time in the future, take a moment to remind yourself of what your fuel filter question is.

Fuel Drop Two: Macro and Micro Nutrients

Fueling the body well becomes more intuitive over time. However, most of us have been exposed to so many mixed messages over the years, that it's helpful to ground ourselves in the basics. Let's talk about what macro and micro nutrients are and what foods you'll find them in. To ground ourselves in the basics, let's start with the oxford dictionary definitions of nutrient and nourishment.

- A nutrient is "A substance that provides nourishment essential for growth and the maintenance of life"

- The definition of nourishment is "The food or other substances necessary for growth, health, and good condition".
- The word Macro means large. And the word Micro means small.

While there are different philosophies about the proportions our bodies need, it is generally recognized that there are three main macronutrients. In alphabetical order they are: carbohydrates, fats, and protein. The list of micronutrients is longer, but is generally made up of various vitamins and minerals.

Macronutrient Tripod
Since there are three macronutrients, let's use the visual of a modern camera-tripod. I say modern because most modern camera-tripods have adjustable legs and some level of flexibility to allow for your perfect picture set-up. Can you picture it?

Visualize adjusting the legs of the tripod so you can capture your picture at the perfect angle. Now, assuming you really like your camera, or phone if you use your phone to take picture... what would you say if I suggested balancing your nice camera on two legs instead of three. How comfortable are you with that?

Pretty likely that you'll say "No Way". Would your answer be as confident and as immediate if I asked you how comfortable you are with the idea of fueling your body with two

137

macronutrients instead of three? I'd like to encourage you to think about these three macronutrients using the dictionary definition... *substances that provide nourishment essential for growth and the maintenance of life.*

While foods are often associated with one of the three macronutrients, many are actually a combination. In addition, whole foods contain a variety of micronutrients as well, which is one reason it's so beneficial that we fuel our bodies with whole foods when possible. For example, when we eat one cup of broccoli, we are getting 6 grams of carbohydrates (including 2 grams of dietary fiber), 3 grams of protein, and it is also a source for vitamin C and vitamin K. Let's talk about one more example to really highlight that point. An avocado, which is typically found on a list of dietary fats, is also a source of carbohydrates and protein. In addition, it is a source for a number of vitamins, including folate; and a number of minerals, including potassium.

Hopefully that fuels your motivation to get your nutrients from eating whole foods as often as is possible given your time-budget and your money-budget.

When we were growing up and learning the food pyramid, we often learned to associate certain foods with certain food groups. Can you picture that loaf of bread, slice of bread, and bowl of pasta that usually appeared as the base of most old-school food pyramids? We have some old programing about what a carbohydrate looks like. Are you ready to upgrade your nutrient-to-food-type map? Since all three macronutrients are important, let's talk about them in alphabetical order starting with carbohydrates. For each macronutrient, we'll list some foods by their predominant macronutrient as a tool for upgrading our nutrient-to-food-type map.

Carbohydrates

In this carbohydrate section, in addition to listing foods, I am also going to list food-types. I find that when I organize them into broader food types, it helps balance out that old image of grains as the main source of carbohydrates.

First, I'll list the broader food types with a single food example, and then after that, we'll list some foods.

Non-starchy vegetable carbohydrates
example: spinach

Starchy vegetable carbohydrates
example: sweet potatoes

Fruit carbohydrates
example: blueberries

Legume carbohydrates
example: chick peas

Grain carbohydrates
example: rice

Non-starchy vegetables

I'll list three, then you can list a few, and then I'll list some more. Kale, Asparagus, Broccoli. Your turn.

Here's a list of some non-starchy vegetable carbohydrates (including those first three so you have them all in one place):

Asparagus
Bok Choy
Broccoli
Brussel Sprouts
Cauliflower
Celery
Collards
Cucumber
Green Beans
Kale
Parsley
Spinach
Zucchini

Starchy vegetables
   Carrots
   Sweet Potatoes

What other starchy vegetables come to mind?

_____ _____

_____ _____

_____ _____

Here's a list of some starchy vegetable carbohydrates:

Beets

Carrots

Sweet Potatoes

White Potatoes

Winter Squashes (i.e. butternut squash)

Yams

Fruit carbohydrates

Starting with the lower glycemic fruit:

Berries

Lemon and Lime

Grapefruit and Oranges

Apples and Pears

The sweeter and higher glycemic fruits:

Bananas

Mangoes

Dates

There are many more fruits to choose from. If you are interested in reading more about their nutritional content, *Self* has a great nutrition facts tool. To help you find it easily, we have a link to it from our "tools" section at FueltheBodyWell.com.

Legumes

What comes to mind for you when you hear legumes?

Here's a list of some legumes:

Black beans

Garbanzo Beans (also known as chick peas)

Lentils

Lima beans

Peanuts

Peas

Grains

Buckwheat (also known as kasha)

Oatmeal

Rice

Rye and other Cereal Grains

Wheat

Dietary Fats

Dietary fats support our bodies in staying satiated and so much more. We'll start with the mighty avocado. A slice or 2 of avocado makes for a terrific long-lasting snack.

Sources of dietary fat include:

Avocado

Chia seeds

Coconut

(The coconut meat. Not the coconut water, which is a carbohydrate)

Nut butters

Olives

Raw nuts (for example almonds, cashews, and walnuts)

Raw seeds (for example pumpkin and sunflower seeds)

Protein

Some of the foods we already listed are a source of protein as well as the macronutrient they are listed under. For example, one ounce of pepitas (which are seeds) has 7 grams of protein. One cup of peas has 8 grams of protein.

To kick off our list of proteins, I'll start with a couple of the most recognized plant forms of protein: soy (for example tofu and tempeh), pea protein, and hemp protein powder. If you are going to get all your protein from plant sources, be mindful of where you are getting your B vitamins.

Now let's talk about the animal forms of protein. Top of the list for me these days has been sardines. I never thought I'd like them, but my husband convinced me to try them. and it was worth it. Sardines are packed full of protein, healthy fats, carbohydrates, and a beautiful serving of vitamin D, vitamin B12, calcium, and selenium.

Other animal proteins include eggs, fish, fowl, and meat. If you do eat animal protein, as much as your time-budget and money-budget allow for, pay attention to the source of where those foods are coming from and how they are raised. The level of nutrients in your food is directly related to the quality of the food. If you are eating an animal protein and that animal was fed low quality food or fed food that you have food sensitivities to, that could impact how nourishing it will be for your body.

Nutrient-to-food-type map

Now that we have listed some foods by their predominant macronutrient, what are you noticing about your nutrient-to-food-type map? What stands out for you as you think back on fuel drop two?

Fuel Drop Three:
What Fuels YOUR Body Well

The reason there are so many different eating methodologies out there is because everyone is a little bit different. Yes, we have many similarities, which means general guidelines can apply to many. However, when we get into specific meal plans, or specific proportions of the three macronutrients, that's when we can best see how one plan can work for someone and not for someone else.

If you've read more than one nutrition or diet book, you've probably noticed that the theories from one to another can be conflicting. Don't lose heart! That's actually liberating information. Why? In a sense, it is a call to each of us to feel empowered. Since currently, there is no conclusive and definitive scientific evidence for how each specific individual should be fueling their body for optimal wellness, what we can do is start with the science that is available and from there, look within.

Looking within assumes we can hear the messages that our body and our inner wisdom are trying to communicate with us, which is why this chapter about nourishing foods comes in the later part of your Guidebook. Notice all the ways you've deepened your connection with your inner wisdom chapter by chapter, fuel drop by fuel drop. Notice all the static you've cleared out. We've already explored our food choices from a meta perspective. We've upgraded our self-talk. We've paid attention to those Zappers, such as foods that interrupt our connection between our innate wisdom and our decision making. We learned how to notice if we have any food sensitivities that are unique to our bodies. We've built a strong foundation for being able to partner with our inner wisdom to notice what fuels OUR bodies well. Then, we grounded ourselves in the basics about macro and micro nutrients.

Take a moment to reflect back to the beginning of the Guidebook and notice the ways you have deepened your connection with your inner wisdom since then. Notice all the tools you have, all the fuel drops you can reach for. These tools will support you as you look within to know what fuels your body well. Here are 5 tips to remind you of how much you already know about fueling your body well:

1. Eat well balanced meals using the best ingredients you have available to you based on your schedule, the time of year, your location, and your budget.
2. Give your system time to digest between meals.
3. Avoid chemicalized foods since they can disrupt your body's innate wisdom.

4. Fuel your body in a loving and respectful manner
5. Number five we'll be talking about in more detail in the next chapter... move your body regularly

Fuel Drop Review

Now that we've talked about Nourishing Foods, let's review our fuel drops:

Fuel Drop One: Food As Fuel
Fuel Drop Two: Macro and Micro Nutrients
Fuel Drop Three: What Foods Fuel YOUR Body Well

In the next chapter, we'll be talking about movement. When we move regularly, we are supporting our bodies as they work to keep our hormones and personal bio-chemistry in balance, which is another great way we can fuel our bodies well.

Key Take-aways
Nourishing Foods

Fuel Drop One: Food As Fuel

- I will aim to think about food as fuel for my beautiful human vehicle
- I will aim to stay curious, observant, and radically honest with myself about the food choices I make
- I will aim to ask myself my fuel filter question

Fuel Drop Two: Macro and Micro Nutrients

- I will aim to eat whole foods some or most of the time since they are a great source of macronutrients as well as a variety of micronutrients
- I will aim to nourish myself with the "macronutrient tripod" which includes: carbohydrates, fats, and proteins
- I will be mindful of my nutrient-to-food-type map and remember that there are many sources of carbohydrates

Fuel Drop Three:
What Foods Fuel YOUR Body Well

- I listen to my inner wisdom
- Some or most of the time I eat well balanced meals using the best ingredients I have available to me based on my schedule, the time of year, my location, and my budget
- Some or most of the time I avoid chemicalized foods since they can disrupt my body's innate wisdom

Chapter Ten
Movement

Movement can be a tool for how we look, and it is also so much more than that. When we move our bodies regularly, we are supporting our bodies as they work to keep our hormones and personal bio-chemistry in balance.

When we only focus on how we look, we zoom all of our attention on the outside of our bodies; but when we also focus on our wellness, we are expanding our love to the inside of our bodies and we are fueling our thoughts and driving our actions in a way that leads us to shine from the inside, out.

The three fuel drops are:

Fuel Drop One: Why Move
Fuel Drop Two: Workout Portions
Fuel Drop Three: Recovery is Part of the Workout

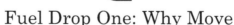

Fuel Drop One: Why Move

Often times, movement is associated with a workout program and a lot of times, in addition to being associated with a workout program, it's associated with helping us fit into our favorite jeans. It's helpful for us to be aware of our focus. When we also focus on being loving to the insides of our bodies, we are leading ourselves to shine from the inside, out. Looking good in our clothes can be a natural extension of being loving to ourselves and certainly a fun side-benefit, but we can have that PLUS **abundant energy** when we focus on shining from the inside.

There are a lot of ways we can move our bodies. Whether you already love fitness or you experience a less enthusiastic reaction when you start to think about movement, do your best to keep your ears open and focused on these movement fuel drops. There is something here for you, aim to find it. Seek to notice and embrace that one distinction that will further your wellness path even more.

Our beautiful human vehicles thrive with regular movement. Whether you choose to skip, swim, or dance your heart out to your favorite song in the privacy of your living room .... whether you choose to lift weights or to park your car an extra block away from your destination so you can fit some extra steps into your day... whatever it is you choose, I'd love to encourage you to try to move your body every single day. Regular physical activity is an important tool for maintaining wellness.

Even if you only have five minutes to do it,
five minutes is better than zero minutes.
Don't let the start stop you.

When we move our bodies regularly, we are supporting them as they work to keep our hormones and personal bio-chemistry in balance. Movement supports your immune system, it helps regulate hormones, curb cravings, it helps clear thinking, supports digestion, better and more restful sleep, and so much more.

The medical benefits

According to Dr. Daniel Amen, a leading authority on brain health, exercise increases your brain's ability to regulate insulin and sugar, maintaining blood-sugar stability. Dr. Amen also says that physical activity reduces cravings for addictive foods like sugary sweets and high-calorie, high-fat food. It helps you manage stress by immediately lowering stress hormones, and it makes you more resistant to stress over time. And engaging in exercise on a routine basis normalizes melatonin production in the brain and improves sleeping habits.

Need more reasons?

According to Dr. Pamela Peeke, who is a woman with an extensive list of credentials to her name including New York Times bestselling author and Pew Scholar in nutrition and metabolism, physical activity increases the prefrontal connections in our brains, and that helps us make better decisions that override those hormone-driven cues.

What are some of the other benefits of movement? They are numerous! See how many you can think of right now.

Here are a few from Dr. Christiane Northrup, who has been an incredible voice for women's wellness for decades.

- Better immune system functioning
- Less depression and anxiety
- Better mental efficiency and speed
- More relaxation and more enthusiasm
- Stronger bones
- More restful sleep
- Decreased insulin sensitivity
- More energy
- Weight control

How does that sound? Pretty great, right? I hope knowing some of the many ways that regular movement supports you in Being Well is a great motivation to move your body.

Reluctance and Motivation

The root cause of reluctance to workout is different for each of us. What I am going do is talk about two common reasons. As you read, allow the examples to stimulate your inner-exploration. Notice what comes up for you. Notice what resonates and notice what other thoughts and ideas come in.

Aptitude

One common reason for workout reluctance is that sometimes people just don't feel like they are good at it. In a conversation I recently had with my friend Laura, we were talking about working out and she said to me "I've never been good at it. I still remember how much I hated gym in elementary school, I wasn't ever any good at it."

By the time we get to elementary school, we've had a lot of experience at some thing. Playtime meant different things for each of us when we were small. Some of us climbed jungle gyms, some of us spent time listening to music, some of us played board games and some of us spent time with finger paints. We all arrived at elementary school with different experiences. If you were watching other kids that were seemingly more coordinated than you in elementary school gym class, it very possibly means they had more years of experience than you did.

If at that moment that you felt unsure, someone had encouraged you to keep trying, is it possible that you would have gotten better? What would your belief about movement be as an adult if you knew that everyone had to practice their way into getting better? It's never too late to start. There are studies on older adults, which demonstrate measurable benefits to starting a workout program even in mature adulthood. For example, Tufts University did a study where postmenopausal women did just two days a week of progressive strength training and the results were increased strength and increased bone density.

Not enough time
Another common reason for workout reluctance is time. Sometimes we hold a belief that if we don't have time for a full workout, then there is no point in working out at all. If you can, remember that five minutes is better than zero minutes. Also keep in mind that there are some really great workouts you can do in ten minutes. You can even park just a little further from your destination (assuming it's safe to do so) and get a little extra walking in that way.

What language motivates you?

If you are already feeling reluctant to workout, then it will be important that you speak to yourself in a language that you will respond to. Are you motivated by accomplishing certain goals? Are you motivated by avoiding certain situations? In the book *Personality Language*, Dr. Wyatt Woodsmall and his wife Marilyne Woodsmall write that 50% of us are predominantly "moving towards" people, meaning, we are more often motivated by what we want and the other 50% of us are predominantly "moving away from" people, meaning we are often more motivated by avoiding the things we don't want.

If I say the words achieve or accomplish, what thoughts and feelings come to mind? What if I say the words avoid or steer clear of, are the thoughts that surfaced different? What language motivates you, moving towards or a moving away? Talk to yourself in the way that will motivate YOU.

Fuel Drop Two: Workout Portions

A well-balanced workout helps us prioritize how to spend our limited time-budget to get the most out of any time we spend working out.

If you are too busy to even think about movement right now, let this plant a seed for you because one day you will be in a place that you have the time-budget to allow for movement. Until then, remember that 5-minutes is way better than zero minutes, so do what you can without "shoulding" all over yourself.

Workout Buckets

In order to talk about portions, we first need to talk about ways we can group workout types. Once we group our movement into workout types, then we'll be able to think about portions and about well-balanced movement. (Just like we aim to think about well-balanced meals!) Let's think of these groups as buckets or containers for organizing various types of movement.

Is there one and only one way to group workout types? No, there isn't. There are many philosophies and many experts in movement, but no single definitive workout protocol that works for each and every one of us because we are each similar, and we are also each unique. Our bodies were designed to move. The how and the how often are unique to each of us, which is a wonderful opportunity for us to connect with ourselves.

Allow that to remind you that YOU are the expert of you. Use the data and studies that are available to inform you. And certainly, if you have any questions or any doubts, consult your healthcare practitioner.

35 Years of Experience

I have been a recreational athlete for 35 years and counting. Over the years, I have earned a number of accolades from competing and more importantly, I have remained injury-free for the vast majority of that time. These workout buckets distill those 35 years of experience, plus the many books and published studies I've read on the topic, into an organized, easy-to-navigate methodology. There are so many workout trends that it is sometimes challenging for people to know which workout to do and how to best invest our precious time. My solution for that is to organize workouts into groups and then balance workout portions.

The Buckets

First I'll list my workout buckets, and then we'll cover each one. Once we've organized workout types, we'll be able to think about portions and about well-balanced movement.

1. Body in Motion
2. Pelvic Floor Strength
3. Total Body Strength Training
4. Cardio
5. Flexibility
6. Mobility & Balance
7. Breath

If you are new to fitness and that sounds like a long list, take a deep breath and remind yourself that we start with one step and then we take another and one day, looking back we can be amazed at how far we've come. Allow yourself to build a foundation and give yourself permission to celebrate every time you move your body with loving intentions.

If you are a seasoned recreational athlete, you may be wondering why I didn't include more categories. To that I'd say that most activities can be neatly organized into one of these 8 categories. For example, core work can be done as part of strength training or as part of cardio depending on what you are doing to work your core.

The Seven Workout Buckets

1. Body in Motion

Body in Motion includes all the small choices we make each day. If we park our cars a little bit further from the destination so we can get in a little bit of extra walking. If we ride our bikes for fun around the block, or if we ride our bike with purpose as our mode of transportation.

Body in Motion means being cognizant of your posture as you are sitting, standing, or walking throughout your day. Body in Motion includes dancing in the privacy of our living room to our favorite song. Body in Motion includes taking a walk with friends to connect and catch up. What else could body in motion mean in your life?

What we track and measure we are more likely to notice, and what we notice, we are more likely to take action on. Do you think you'd be up for jotting down a little note for yourself and record what Body in Motion activities you do over the next week?

2. Pelvic Floor Strength

Before we dive any further into this particular workout bucket, I want to give you a heads up that we will be talking about our female anatomy during this one workout type.

Our pelvic floor muscles can be out of sight, out of mind, but peeing in your pants is no fun. Statistics are not on our side as we age if we don't strengthen those muscles. It's worth it to give some attention to your pelvic floor strength now. These are the muscles that control continence (that's bladder AND bowel). Can you see how your body would benefit from giving these muscles a few minutes of focus on a regular basis?

One well-known technique for strengthening your pelvic floor muscles is the kegel. I am going to share some tips right now, but if you are interested in learning more, I'd encourage you to check out Amy Stein, MPT who is a well-recognized expert on this topic.

Tip #1: Acknowledge the laws of gravity
If you are new to kegels, try by starting on your back. As Mickey Marie Morrison describes in her book, Baby Weight, the easiest position for beginners is lying down, where gravity has less effect. You can work your way up to sitting, standing, and maybe eventually even squatting as you develop strength and control.

Tip #2: Clench and Relax
The kegel exercise happens during the act of clenching and the unclenching. Both are important.

Tip #3: Be kind and patient with yourself
Most of us are more likely to do something if we see the benefit and we are even more likely to stick with it if we are good at it. Hopefully by now you can see the benefits of strengthening your pelvic floor.

Now here's the bad news, it takes most people a lot of practice. Doesn't it seem like something we should just be able to do? If you are among the few that find it easy, count yourself lucky. For the rest of us, my best advice is to take one day at a time. Once you have the hang of them and you are more confident that you are getting the correct muscles, you can do them discreetly anywhere. At a stoplight, waiting in line... there are so many resourceful little ways you can squeeze in your kegels. (pun intended!) Even if you can only allocate one minute here and there, those 'one minutes' will make a difference over time

3. Total Body Strength Training

The 3rd workout type is Strength Training. I resisted incorporating strength training into my routine for a surprisingly long time given what I know about the benefits. I resisted because even though I knew logically it wouldn't be possible, I held onto an irrational concern that if I lifted weights I'd end up looking like a young Arnold Schwarzenegger. If you are feeling resistant, I completely empathize.

Strength training is incredibly important for women, especially as we age. It matters for our bone density and it matters so we can prevent muscle loss. It has also been shown to provide an increase in metabolic rate, which is super-helpful for weight loss and long-term weight control.

The average adult loses muscle each year. Muscles are a use it or lose it. Which means that disuse leads to muscle loss. Ready for the good news? According to multiple sources, including the

Tufts study I mentioned earlier, strength training 2-3 days per week is one of the best ways to keep muscles healthy and strong. Done regularly, strength training builds bone and muscle to preserve strength and energy. Are you feeling motivated to incorporate strength training 2-3 days per week?

4. Cardio

Cardio is a common term used to refer to workouts that provide cardiovascular conditioning. This "cardio" category is a catchall for workouts like aerobics, marching in place, running, swimming, cycling, hiking, jumping rope, dance class, spin class, playing soccer, HIIT training- which is high intensity interval training, and so much more. There are a lot of options for cardiovascular conditioning, so choose one that is right for your current level and build your way into fitness.

If you ever find yourself less enthusiastic about your cardio, consider exploring options until you find one that you enjoy. When you do start to explore and try out different cardio workouts, one piece of advice I'd like to give you is not to be intimidated if you don't know the lingo for a certain workout. Remember, everyone was new at some point so don't let the start stop you.

An important thing about this cardio bucket is to differentiate this bucket from the *Body in Motion* bucket. If you are out for a leisurely walk, that's usually going to be Body in Motion. Even if you are on the elliptical or the stationary bike going at a nice easy pace, if you can chat with friends or read, that's likely *Body in Motion* also. How will you know if your workout is a cardio workout? Check your heart rate. Or do a talk

160

test. If you can still sing a song or carry on a long conversation without any breathlessness, you are most likely in the *Body in Motion* bucket. The *Body in Motion* bucket is important, just be aware of which bucket you are in because they are different buckets for a reason.

Looking for some cardio motivation?
- According to the American Heart Association, moderate-to-vigorous exercise improves your overall cardiovascular health.
- According to the Cleveland Clinic, aerobic exercise can decrease risk of heart disease, lower blood pressure, increase HDL or "good" cholesterol, help better control blood sugar, assist in weight management or weight loss, and improve lung function.

Plus, in my experience, I've noticed that a lot of people find that including cardio as a part of their workout portions seems to really help elevate their mood. I know that's true for me. I love being happy. What about you?

5. Flexibility and 6. Mobility & Balance

The next two workout types we are going to talk about are the 5th bucket, which is flexibility and the 6th bucket, which is mobility and balance.

Flexibility can include stretching and foam rolling. Yoga fits well into both the flexibility and balance (and more buckets too depending on which style you are practicing). In addition to yoga, another balance and mobility workout is Tai Chi. If you are interested in reading a book on mobility, *The Supple Leopard* by Kelly Starrett is a thorough resource.

Balance and mobility are important and here's why... If you are a 'moving towards' person, you may want to think about this *Mobility and Balance* bucket as moving with grace and ease. If you are a 'moving away from' person, you may want to think about it as moving without pain or as not falling.

7. Breath
Oxygen is ESSENTIAL to our wellness. Use breath as a tool to fuel your body well. It's free (at least it is now and for the foreseeable future), and it doesn't take up a lot of time. The return on your time investment is so huge. Breathe on purpose and often, and know you are doing something wonderful for yourself.

If our goal is Vibrant Vitality and long-term wellness, then recovery is a MUST. We'll talk about recovery more in Fuel Drop Three. That wraps up our 7 buckets and sets us up to talk about workout portions.

Workout Portions
How do we measure if the workout portions are well balanced? When it comes to the proportions of your portions, that will be individual based on your current fitness level and time budget, but here's a guideline for you.... If it feels right for your body, your current fitness level, and your time budget, aim

to fit in 3 or more of these buckets over the course of a two-week time period. If you can do more, great. If you can't carve out the time right now, just take a deep breath and remind yourself that five minutes is better than zero minutes.

As you are experimenting with what portions work best for you, be patient with yourself. Stay conscious about your choices and be kind to yourself along the path. Remember, wellness is a journey and sometimes it's easiest when you take one step at a time and keep yourself pointed in the direction of your true north. In the day-to-day it's sometimes harder to see what we WILL be able to see in time when we look back.

Fuel Drop Three: Recovery Is Part Of The Workout

If our goal is Vibrant Vitality and long-term wellness, then recovery is a must. Recovery is it's own fuel drop for a reason. Notice, it is not part of the workout buckets, even though it could easily and logically be organized that way. Does that help drive in for you just how important recovery is for your wellness? This isn't a long fuel drop, but it's an important one.

Whether you want to call it rest, repair, rejuvenation, or recovery if you are moving your body regularly, build this into your plan. Recovery can take many forms.

Here are some examples:

- getting a full night sleep
- taking a nice bath
- maybe even getting a massage
- active recovery (for example, a mobility workout)
- building in a rest day every week (which would be a day with no cardio or strength training)
- a strategically planned week off from cardio and strength training every so often, for example a week off every 6-8 weeks.

The goal of all of this, both the movement and the recovery, is to take really good care of your wonderful and loyal human vehicle. Remember to be kind to yourself along the way, it's a process. We are exactly where we are. The question is, are we making the choices that lead us to where we want to go.

Fuel Drop Review

Now that we've talked about Movement, let's review our fuel drops:

Fuel Drop One: Why Move
Fuel Drop Two: Workout Portions
Fuel Drop Three: Recovery is Part of the Workout

Here's wishing you joyful and effortless movement that furthers you on your wellness path!

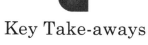

Key Take-aways
Movement

Movement can be a tool for how we look, and it is also so much more than that; it is a tool for supporting our overall wellness. When we focus on how we look, we zoom all of our attention on the outside of our bodies. When we also focus on our wellness, we are expanding our love for the inside of our bodies and we are fueling our thoughts and driving our actions in a way that leads us to shine from the inside, out.

Fuel Drop One: Why Move

- I aim to move regularly so I can support and partner with my body to regulate my personal bio-chemistry and so much more
- Even if I only have five minutes to move, I know that five minutes is better than zero minutes

Fuel Drop Two: Workout Portions

- When I do have time to budget for movement, I will aim to consider balancing my workout portions to include more than one workout type
- The seven workout buckets are: Body in Motion, Pelvic Floor Strength, Total Body Strength Training, Cardio, Flexibility, Mobility & Balance, Breath
- I will aim to remember that what I track and measure I am more likely to notice and take action on

Fuel Drop Three: Recovery is Part of the Workout

- I will aim to be kind to myself along the way and aim to build recovery into my movement practice
- I will keep in mind that the goal is to take really good care of my wonderful and loyal human vehicle

Chapter Eleven
Building The Fuel Drop Framework

You've just built a sturdy and powerful foundation one fuel drop at a time, and now this is where it all comes together.

Stacking the Fuel Drops

What we are going to do now is list all of the fuel drops one at a time. As you read through the list of fuel drops, notice which resonate with you the most. If this is your second time reading the Guidebook (or more), you may find that the fuel drops that resonate most may change over time or they may be the same each time. Notice that because either way, it's information for you.

All of the Fuel Drops

1. Know Your True North
2. Know Why
3. Remind Yourself Often
4. Our *Meta* Food Choices
5. Presentness In Our Meals
6. Post-meal Rituals
7. External Messages
8. Internal Self Talk
9. Our Wellness 5
10. Zappers
11. The Messages In Cravings
12. Mood Altering And Addictive Substances
13. Nourishing Our Cells
14. Nourishing Our Hearts

The 5 Daily Basics
A-W-E-Z-Z awesome, awesome, awesome are we.

A for air. Fueling our cells with oxygen

W for water. Being hydrated

E for energy. Harmonizing our Energy Flow

Z for zone. Honoring the digestion zone.

Z ZZZ's. Rest and rejuvenation.

The Power of Repetition

Now what we are going to do is amp up the benefits even more. I am going to ask you a series of question so you can deepen what you learned and benefit from this experience long after you finish reading this book. As you are answering these questions, remember to be kind to yourself. You may not have immediate answers to all of these questions and that is completely ok. Even if you don't recall the answer immediately,

168

the act of lovingly searching with no self-judgment will bring up something you can benefit from. As you read these questions, allow your mind to think back to the fuel drop and retrieve the information:

What is your true north?

Have you had the opportunity yet to be in a situation that in the past you would have made one set of choices, and since having started the Guidebook, you have made a different set of choices?

What elements from the 5 Daily Basics have you tried?

Have you had a situation come up yet that you were able to partner with your body and use one of these tools rather than experiencing energy-zapping stress?

Have you ever found yourself remembering your AWE double Z's, thinking about taking a deep, cell nourishing breath, and then telling yourself you didn't have time? What will you do when you are in that situation next time?

Can you think of one or two tools for supporting Presentness in your meals?

What is your typical post-meal routine?

What record is playing in the background for you? Are your go-to messages the same or different than they were before you started?

Who are your Wellness 5?

What were some of the Wellness Blockers that were on your path in the past? What counter zappers have you used to face them?

Have you had any food cravings? If so, did you have an opportunity to decipher the message in your cravings?

What have you done in the last week to nourish your heart?

Have you had the opportunity to experience the benefit of additional rest and rejuvenation (and if that was not possible yet, have you made some aspirational rest and rejuvenation goals?)

Have you uncovered any food sensitivities?

What do the terms happy belly and wellness-welcoming terrain bring to mind?

Have you experienced any moments where your shifting hormones felt like a tumultuous sea? If so, were you able to reach for your fuel drops to navigate back to wellness?

Have you taken a moment to feel really proud of your wonderful and complex female body?

What does your fuel flower look like?

What is your fuel filter question?

How has the food-to-nutrient mapping that we did supported your food choices?

What are some foods that fuel you well? What are some non-food sources of fuel that fill you up?

What are one or two reasons that our beautiful human vehicles thrive with movement?

Choose one of the seven workout types and then notice what activities you have done in the last week in that workout type.

Have you experienced the energy boost from seeing, accepting, and loving more of the hues of your human-ness?

WOHHHOOOO!!!
Congratulations on reaching this milestone!!!!

In the *Integration* chapter, we'll do a couple of exercises because seeing what you've accomplished can be another tool for fueling your forward momentum and furthering your wellness path even more. Are you up for fueling your forward momentum even more?

The Fuel Drop Framework

Your Wellness Destination

- Know Your True North
- Know Why
- Remind Yourself Often

A-W-E-Z-Z

- Air (breath)
- Water (hydration)
- Energy (harmonizing our energy flow)
- Zone (honoring the digestion zone)
- ZZZ's (rest and rejuvenation)

How We Eat Matters

- Our *Meta* Food Choices
- Presentness in our meals
- Post-meal rituals

What Our Minds Are Consuming

- External Messages
- Internal Self Talk
- Our Wellness 5

The Fuel Drop Framework

Wellness Blockers
- Zappers
- The Messages In Cravings
- Mood Altering And Addictive Substances

Human Vehicle Basics
- Nourishing Our Cells
- Nourishing Our Hearts
- Rest And Rejuvenation

Internal Terrain
- Food Sensitivities
- Happy Belly
- Hormones

Nourishing Foods
- Food As Fuel
- Macro And Micro Nutrients
- What Foods Fuel YOUR Body Well

Movement
- Why Move
- Workout Portions
- Recovery is part of the Workout

Chapter Twelve
Integration

Think about your wellness as a cozy room for just a moment. As you picture your cozy room - what's there? Is there a comfy couch or chair to sit in to enjoy the view? What else is in the room? What does the amazing view look like? Remember, this is completely for fun so you can have a made up landscape. You can have beach AND meadows with wild flowers, you can have sunshine AND stars. You can have a blue sky with fluffy white clouds, or you may even choose a lavender sky with golden streaks.

Nestled in your cozy room, what's the perfect temperature for you? Do you like to feel a little bit warm so you can open the window and smell the fresh air from your beautiful view? Or maybe you like it a little bit crisp so you can be wrapped in a blanket. What's comfortable for you? Can you picture it? Are you comfortable? Are you nice and cozy and enjoying your view?

What would happen if the temperature in your cozy room changes by half of a degree? Would you still be able to enjoy the serene moment? What if your cozy room changes by 10 or 20 degrees. Do you think that would have a different impact than the half of a degree change? Would it distract you from enjoying the cozy room? Would it distract you from enjoying the view?

Do you want to go back to your perfect temperature? Go ahead, picture it again. Picture it the way you want it.

Our Wellness Set Point

We all have a set-point where we are comfortable. Whether it's in our fun filled imagination, or it's in our real life. Whether we are talking about the temperature outside or the weight on our bathroom scale or our level of energy and vitality or our dress size. Isn't it true that you have set points where you are comfortable? What are some of your set points?

What insight does that give you about set points and personal expectations? One thing I hope it does is help you see that when we expect amazing, for example, when we expect our wonderful cozy room with the amazing view to be the way we want it, we create a set point with our expectations.

What expectations do you have about your wellness? What have you expected about your wellness set point in the past, and more importantly, what do you want your new wellness set point to be? You may want to capture some of your thoughts by writing them down.

While I'd like to be able to say that now that you have your new wellness set-point and the tools of the full framework, the wellness journey will be forever perfect . . . but I can only say that if we define perfect. A perfectly present and fully lived life comes with lots of color, lots of zigs, and lots of zags. Perfect might even mean unexpected and potentially uninvited opportunities to practice your fuel drops. If you can, remember that any obstacles or challenges you face on your path to your true north are part of the adventure then you'll be even further on your path towards effortless wellness.

The Power of Questions

Take a moment right now to think of one possible scenario of what could come up for you and how you'll use these tools to continue zigging and zagging in the direction of your true north.

What was your situation? What tools did you use? How confident are you that you'll remember to use those tools if that situation occurs? How confident are you that if you forget to use the tools at first, that you will eventually remember to use the tools?

Are you predominantly a moving towards person or a moving away from person? Knowing that, are there any additional tools you want to plan for?

Was your answer the same? Did you add anything?

If one tool doesn't work for you, you have others. Not every tool will work in every situation. And sometimes, even if it's the same situation, there could be other factors that make a different tool more effective. Make sense?

Scenarios Exercise

Answer these questions one by one.

Scenario 1:

Picture what your life would look like next week if you don't use any of the tools or techniques you just learned. What does that look like?

What types of choices are you making? How are you feeling? What's your level of energy?

Now take that same scenario out further... How do you feel next year at this time?

Now, picture yourself five years from now. Can you picture yourself in your day-to-day routines?

Can you picture the types of choices you'll be making?

If you have other people around you - either work colleagues, or loved ones, or children - how are your choices impacting them?

Scenario 2:

Picture your life next week if you implement just one or a few of the fuel drops. What tools will they be?

When and how will you fit them into your day?

What will be the pros and what will be the challenges of fitting those wellness choices into your day?

What types of choices are you making? How are you feeling? What's your level of energy?

Now, take that same scenario out further. How do you feel next year at this time?

When you hit a wellness bump along the journey, did you remember to lean on the fuel drops and/or focus on the 5 Daily Basics? Did you learn from the experience and then continue forward in the direction of your true north?

Are your wellness choices becoming more intuitive?

Have you taken the power of repetition away from the advertisers and applied it to what fuels your body well?

Now, picture yourself five years from now. Can you picture yourself in your day-to-day routines? Can you picture the types of choices you'll be making?

If you have other people around you - either work colleagues, or loved ones, or children - how are your choices impacting them?

Compare and Contrast
How was your life different between scenario 1 and scenario 2?

Having visited two possible versions of your future self, if your future self could give your present self one piece of advice right now, what would it be? Write it down.

_____

_____

_____

Congratulations

I am so happy for you and am deeply honored to have shared a part of your wellness journey with you. I hope you are enjoying your next level of Vibrant Vitality and that you feel confident and prepared for what's next on your wellness path.

If you have any feedback, insights, or experiences that you are up for sharing with me, I'd love to hear from you. The best email for that is Hello@FueltheBodyWell.com

Wishes for abundant wellness, continued Vitality, and may you shine from the inside, out!

Be well,

Simona

Appendix
Applications and Tips for the 5 Daily Basics

The Daily Basics Jumpstart

This is called the Daily Basics Jumpstart to encourage you to do the 5 Daily Basics daily for a few days so you can really learn them. With practice, they take less time and become more effortless. As you are reading about the Daily Basics Jumpstart, you may want to start to visualize yourself doing these steps. Picture where you'll be, visualize the date on the calendar, picture yourself smiling at the end of each day knowing how much progress you are making on your wellness path.

The 5 Daily Basics

A for air. Fueling our cells with oxygen

W for water. Being hydrated

E for energy. Harmonizing our Energy Flow

Z for zone. Honoring the digestion zone.

Z ZZZ's. Rest and rejuvenation.

Let's talk about applications for each of these one at a time starting with A.

A for air, for breath, for oxygen

During the days of you Jumpstart, plan a time each day to breath consciously for one minute. The best way to ensure you make your conscious breathing session happen is to either schedule it on the calendar with a pop-up reminder, or to add it to the beginning or end of a habit you already do every day such as brushing your teeth.

If you have a timer or stopwatch feature on your watch or phone, it would be ideal to use it. One minute can feel like a surprisingly long time when you are first incorporating this daily habit into your routine.

W for water, for hydration

Here are your three water-related assignments during your Daily Basics Jumpstart:

1. Bring a big glass or water bottle of water with you up to bed and leave it bedside. In the morning, start your day by drinking it.

   How much water will you be starting your day with? You can experiment with the amount to figure out what feels right for your body. A great starting place is 10-12 ounces of water.

2. Sip water throughout the day. (You may want to stop in the evening so trips to the bathroom don't interrupt your restful night's sleep).

3. Third is a rule about when NOT to drink water. You may want to consider separating your eating and your hydration. If you need to drink a lot of water with your meals, it may be an indication that you aren't chewing enough. And if you need to "trick" your body into being full by filling it with water during the meal, it may be an indication that you have some room to be in more harmony with yourself and your inner wisdom. If you are up for giving this 3rd hydration rule a try, stop drinking water ten minutes prior to eating, and hold off on water for at least twelve minutes after eating.

Why wait only 12 minutes to drink water?
You can wait longer than 12 minutes. Some sources say to wait 30 minutes so you can keep the pH in your gut the right balance for digestion. The reason the Daily Basics Jumpstart recommendation is 12 minutes is because it's manageable. It's more important to incorporate a tiny habit that gives you most of the benefits and that can integrate into your busy life rather than to try to 'hit it out of the park' with a big new commitment that will be more challenging to maintain for the long haul.

E for Energy and harmonizing our energy flow

For our Daily Basics Jumpstart, aim to do the 3-minute Routine daily. The first few times you do your "3-minute" routine, it may take 7 – 10 minutes to do, but once you've done it a few times, you should be able to complete the full routine in 3 minutes.

The 3-minute Routine

The 3-minute Routine is designed to boost your level of physical energy, support the flow of energy currents in your body, and to communicate to your body when you are experiencing modern stress (vs. running-from-a-bear stress).

The 3-minute Routine includes 6 techniques
1. A Cell-Nourishing Breath
2. Finger Squeeze
3. Stand and Stretch
4. Arm Pretzel
5. Back of Ear Massage
6. Eye Rest

1. A Cell-Nourishing Breath

We start the 3-minute Routine by taking a deep, cell-nourishing breath. Place one hand on your upper abdomen as a tactical queue to remind you to breath deeply. Breathe in through your nose, hold, and breathe out through your mouth. Aim to have the exhale last for longer than the inhale.

Breath is one of our fastest tools to boost our energy. Taking just one deep, cell-nourishing breath can have an immediate impact on our physiology, our emotions, and our mood.

2. Finger Squeeze

Get your circulation and your energy flowing by simply squeezing the ends of each of your fingers and your thumbs on both hands.

188

Many of our meridians start or end in our finger tips, which means by squeezing the ends of our fingers, we are giving ourselves a quick boost. Our heart meridian, our small intestines meridian, our pericardium meridian, our triple warmer meridian, and our lung meridian all either start or end in one of our fingers or thumbs. It's so fast and easy and the return on the time investment is terrific. If you happen to be barefoot, you can also do a toe squeeze too.

3. Stand and Stretch
If you are physically able, stand up and stretch. Stretch your arms up over your head and then clasp your hands. With your hands clasped over your head and your feet planted firmly on the ground, slowly begin to lean to the right by bending at the waist. Then make your way back to the center. From that center position, slowly lean to the left. Then make your way back to center. When you are back in the center position again, see if you can reach even higher. Then slowly let your arms come back down to a relaxed neutral position.

Standing and stretching brings our attention to our breath, our balance, our arms, and our legs. The movement also moves our blood, our energy, and oxygen throughout our bodies circulating nourishment and whisking away toxins.

4. Arm Pretzel

The next two routines (the arm pretzel and the back of ear massage) are both techniques that I learned from Donna Eden. I call this fourth technique the arm pretzel because that's what it feels like to me. She calls it the modified Wayne Cook posture. It's a great tool for unscrambling any scrambled and chaotic energy. That's important because when your energy is scrambled, not only do you feel off, but you can also impact the energy of the people that are around you.

To do the arm pretzel, put your arms out in front of you with your palms facing each other. Your arms will be perpendicular to your body and parallel to the ground. Now turn your hands so the backs of your hands are facing one another. Cross one arm over the other and clasp your hands together. Once your hands are clasped, bring them down then in towards your body. Your elbows will bend as you bring your hands down towards your body and then up towards your heart. When you are in the arm pretzel position, your hands will be clasped near your heart and your elbows will be pointing downward. From this position, take four full breaths. Then slowly and carefully release your arms back down to a relaxed and neutral position.

5. Back of Ear Massage

This fifth technique is my modification of a Donna Eden energy routine called the triple warmer smoothie. You can find the description of her technique in her books *Energy Medicine* and *Energy Medicine for Women*.

190

In this technique, we focus our loving attention on our triple warmer meridian. The triple warmer is the wonderfully protective part of your energy body that takes charge when you are facing a threat. The challenge is, so many of our modern stresses are not true threats to our life, so we need to partner with our triple warmer so it knows we are safe.

You may want to think of this technique like rubbing a baby's back as they go from fighting-against falling asleep into a peaceful and rejuvenating slumber.

Start by placing your index and middle fingers on your temples and massage by pressing down and moving your fingers in a circular motion. Next slowly start working your massaging fingers away from your temples and towards your ears. When you are next to your ear, begin massaging upward then around and down the backs of your ears as you trace behind your ears. When you reach the bottom of your ears, squeeze your earlobe.

7. Eye Rest

In order see, our brains receive signals from our eyes and then interpret those signals. It's a lot of information coming in all the time. By covering your eyes, you are lowering the amount of stimulation you are taking in and giving your brain a moment to rest and recharge.

Sit with your eyes resting in your cupped hands for three slow and full breaths. You can do this by placing your elbows on a desk or table and cupping each of your hands. Rest your head in the palms of your hands by covering each eye... right cupped palm over the right eye, left cupped palm over the left eye. From that position, your fingertips may be able to comfortably rest on your forehead and your thumbs against your temples.

When you are in the position, your eyes should be comfortably in the dark space under your cupped hands. You can close your eyes or keep them open as you rest your sensory input and relax for three breaths.

The first Z is for ZONE. It's about honoring the digestion zone.

During this Daily Basics Jumpstart, I'd like to strongly encourage you to honor the digestion zone. Honoring the digestion zone means giving your body time to digest between meals. To calculate the time between meals, you can find the free Digestion Zone app on iTunes or use these simple steps to calculate how long to wait between meals.

Step 1: Categorize what you eat
Did you eat a snack, a small meal, a hearty meal, or a feast?

Why wait different times for different meal sizes?
Similar to a small load of laundry vs. filling up the whole machine. In general, the larger the meal, the longer it takes to digest.

Step 2: Set the timer
After you eat, set a timer. You can use the Digestion Zone
app or calculate the time yourself as follows.

For the first 12 minutes: food and water fast
Regardless of what you ate (a snack, meal, or feast), the first
12 minutes of the digestion zone are a food and water fast.

After the 12-minutes
After your 12-minute food and water fast, wait an additional
amount of time before eating more food. For example, for a
snack, you'll wait an additional 30 minutes which makes the
Snack DZ time a total of 42 minutes, although 45 minutes
may be easier to remember.

Snack DZ: 45 minutes total
Small Meal DZ: 1 hour total
Hearty Meal DZ: 2 hours total
Feast DZ: 3 hours total

Step 3: Acknowledge how awesome you are
It is logical and obvious that we want to be good to our
bodies. At the same time, it is challenging when we have
such easy access to eating. We no longer have to get a rock
to open the hard outer shell of an almond nut and pull out the
delicious almond in the middle. Now we can simply grab a
handful of almonds. There are pros and challenges to our
modern eating options. Which means, when you follow the
digestion zone you deserve your own pat on the back!

The second Z in A-W-E double Z is for ZZZZ's.

How are you currently prioritizing your sleep? How do you feel when you wake up in the morning? Are you rested? Are you popping out of bed and ready to start the day? Do you have a specific time you go to sleep at night? A specific time you wake up? What about a bedtime ritual or routine?

As part of the Daily Basics Jumpstart, I'd like to encourage you to choose a consistent time you'd like to be in bed each night. If it's possible, aim to get a full night sleep. If a full night sleep is not possible for you right now, consider making it an aspirational goal. In the meantime, can you add 20 additional minutes to the amount of sleep you are currently getting?

Daily Basics Jumpstart Commitment

Are you ready to commit to your Daily Basics Jumpstart? If so, decide how long you want to commit to. Pick the number of days between three and ten days, and do the 5 Daily Basics each day during that time.

There is not usually an "ideal" time to get started, so waiting until that ideal time could inadvertently have a negative impact on your results. The opposite will be true if you go for it immediately. You will be sending a clear message to every part of yourself that you are committed and congruent in your quest for wellness-flow and more vitality in your everyday life. The more you practice the 5 Daily Basics, the faster and more effortless they become. Once you have practiced them, these potent wellness tools become easier to fit into the nooks and crannies of your day.